Translational Neurosonology

Frontiers of Neurology and Neuroscience

Vol. 36

Series Editor

J. Bogousslavsky Montreux

Translational Neurosonology

Volume Editors

A. Alonso Mannheim
M.G. Hennerici Mannheim
S. Meairs Mannheim

22 figures, 6 in color, and 1 table, 2015

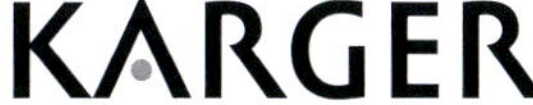

Basel · Freiburg · Paris · London · New York · Chennai · New Delhi · Bangkok · Beijing · Shanghai · Tokyo · Kuala Lumpur · Singapore · Sydney

Frontiers of Neurology and Neuroscience

Vols. 1–18 were published as Monographs in Clinical Neuroscience

PD Dr. Angelika Alonso
Prof. Dr. Michael G. Hennerici
Prof. Dr. Stephen Meairs
Department of Neurology
Universitätsmedizin Mannheim
University of Heidelberg
Theodor-Kutzer-Ufer 1-3
DE–68167 Mannheim (Germany)

Library of Congress Cataloging-in-Publication Data

Translational neurosonology / volume editors, A. Alonso, M.G. Hennerici, S. Meairs.
    p. ; cm. -- (Frontiers of neurology and neuroscience, ISSN 1660-4431 ; vol. 36)
  Includes bibliographical references and indexes.
  ISBN 978-3-318-02790-7 (hard cover : alk. paper) -- ISBN 978-3-318-02791-4 (e-ISBN)
  I. Alonso, A. (Angelika), editor. II. Hennerici, M. (Michael), editor. III. Meairs, Stephen P. (Stephen Philip), 1952- , editor. IV. Series: Frontiers of neurology and neuroscience ; v. 36. 1660-4431
  [DNLM: 1. Nervous System Diseases--ultrasonography. 2. Nervous System--ultrasonography. 3. Translational Medical Research. 4. Vascular Diseases--ultrasonography. W1 MO568C v.36 2015 / WL 141]
  RC349.U47
  616.8'047543--dc23

                                          2014038454

Bibliographic Indices. This publication is listed in bibliographic services, including Current Contents® and Index Medicus.

© Copyright 2015 by S. Karger AG, P.O. Box, CH-4009 Basel (Switzerland)
www.karger.com
Printed in Germany on acid-free and non-aging paper (ISO 9706) by Kraft Druck, Ettlingen
ISSN 1660–4431
e-ISSN 1662–2804
ISBN 978–3–318–02790–7
e-ISBN 978–3–318–02791–4

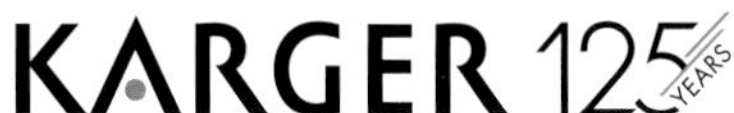

Contents

Preface

Since the introduction of non-invasive ultrasound technologies in clinical practice in the early 1970s, the diagnosis and treatment of neurovascular diseases have made tremendous progress. Today, ultrasound is capable not only of monitoring the early silent stages of atherogenesis in infancy and atherosclerosis in very old age in an increasingly ageing population but also of identifying and evaluating the morphological patterns of plaque development and prognosis during progression and regression in most large arteries of the body. In addition, perfusion studies can be performed to assess arteriolar and capillary networks as well as collateral capacities in small vessel disease.

The ability of ultrasound to visualise both arterial and venous blood flow characteristics, including turbulence vortices and tortuosities, as well as vessel wall structures, thrombus formation and the generation of emboli during treatment or spontaneous fragmentation can be observed and quantified based on circulating microemboli. Translational studies have contributed to increasingly enormous knowledge about the underlying pathomechanisms and molecular biological processes. In line with other vascular imaging modalities, such as magnetic resonance angiography and computed tomography angiograms, vascular ultrasound studies are important tools in individual patients during follow-up. Indeed, ultrasound has become the stethoscope of the stroke physician and has widely replaced palpitation and auscultation in vascular medicine.

In addition, ultrasound has been implemented in prospective randomised clinical trials, both in epidemiological and in interventional studies. The standardisation of examination procedures and refined states of technology and data analysis has helped to identify new pathways for the best medical management of patients, e.g. lifestyle modification; treatment of the risk factors of atherosclerosis and thromboembolism; or interventional and surgical management, such as thrombectomies, stenting and dilatation. In addition, although not yet established in clinical practice, sonothrombolysis with or without drug application has made considerable progress. Catheter-based transcutaneous and intraarterial ultrasounds show enhancement of fibrinolytic agents, and in the early 20th century, the first clinical studies evaluated the adjunct effect of ultrasound in treating patients with acute ischaemic stroke, whether frank insonation of large vessels or by microbubble-enhanced thrombolysis with or without encapsulated tissue plasminogen activator was used.

The transport of microbubbles incorporating other drugs has been tested and is currently being developed to pass through the intact blood-brain barrier (BBB) in specific focused areas, sometimes combined with other neuroimaging technologies for the treatment of non-vascular diseases. Apart from the temporary destruction of the BBB, the closure of vascular leakage may be useful in patients suffering from intracerebral haemorrhage. Increasing knowledge also suggests that ultrasound may be applied for transient focal opening or closure of the BBB if combined with high-resolution MR imaging of brain tissue to facilitate 'microscopic' treatment; with very limited tissue damage, minimally invasive permanent or transient tissue modulation may be achieved, as recently shown for the treatment of essential tremor, Parkinson's disease and other brain disorders.

Animal models and randomised clinical trials are important tools in translational studies, contributing to our increasing knowledge, and will be reviewed in several sections in this book. New developments in technology and imaging refinement will be addressed in addition to supportive technologies used for neurovascular studies; a separate chapter deals with potential bioeffects and safety issues. New aspects of structural and functional imaging will be addressed based on useful information from experimental studies, leading to refined assessment of healthy subjects and of patients with cerebrovascular and neurodegenerative diseases. Finally, recently developed strategies will be presented for non-invasive ultrasound treatment, which is still limited in clinical application but ready to undergo properly designed trial evaluation.

Michael G. Hennerici, Mannheim

Alonso A, Hennerici MG, Meairs S (eds): Translational Neurosonology.
Front Neurol Neurosci. Basel, Karger, 2015, vol 36, pp 1–10 (DOI: 10.1159/000366222)

Principles of Cerebral Ultrasound Contrast Imaging

Jeff Powers[a] · Michalakis Averkiou[b]

[a]Philips Ultrasound, MS 1010, Bothell, Wash., USA; [b]Biomedical Engineering Program, Department of Mechanical Engineering, University of Cyprus, Nicosia, Cyprus

Abstract

Ultrasound contrast is gaining acceptance worldwide as an adjunct to conventional ultrasound imaging. It has clinical applications as diverse as liver disease detection and characterization, myocardial perfusion and wall motion studies, and imaging of cerebral vascularity and perfusion. This paper will focus on imaging techniques used for transcranial ultrasound contrast imaging. The interaction of ultrasound with the microbubbles in the contrast agent is complex and nonlinear. This has led to the development of a variety of imaging modes to improve contrast detection compared with non-contrast optimized modes. This article presents several of these imaging methods in such a way as to help users of ultrasound contrast in the clinic and in research to understand this rapidly developing field.

Introduction

CT and MR imaging modalities have long used intravenously injected contrast material to visualize blood flow in the microcirculation and in larger vessels. Ultrasound has traditionally used Doppler techniques, relying on the motion of blood in arteries and veins, to measure blood flow in larger vessels. However, the low velocities in small vessels coupled with the weak signal from red blood cells puts a lower limit on the velocity detection capability of Doppler techniques. In addition, the patient-to-patient variability of the temporal bone window has limited the widespread adoption of Doppler techniques in transcranial applications.

The use of microbubble-based ultrasound contrast agents (UCAs) enables ultrasound to complement CT and MR in a number of clinical areas in which sensitivity is reduced by inadequate bone windows or in which perfusion is an important clinical differentiator. The portability and real-time nature of ultrasound combined with contrast holds promise for acute stroke patients in an emergency situation. The low cost and the lack of ionizing radiation make ultrasound ideal for monitoring neurology patients during and after therapeutic interventions.

The past three decades have seen the active development of stabilized microbubbles capable of transpulmonary passage for left-side blood pool enhancement by several major pharmaceutical companies [1, 2]. During the same time period, enhancements of ultrasound equipment have provided researchers with the ability to visualize microbubbles within the parenchyma of the liver, kidney, brain, and other organs following an intravenous injection [3–5]. This paper outlines these technological improvements. It begins with a brief review of ultrasound physics to help to clarify how these new imaging developments work and then describes novel imaging techniques as well as other features that complement them that are unique to UCAs.

It must be noted here that to date, no contrast agents have received approval from the Food and Drug Administration for radiological or neurological applications in the United States. In Europe, Canada, and Asia, however, contrast agents have been approved for both cardiology and radiology. This paper is intended to help those involved with ultrasound contrast research to understand this continually evolving field.

Ultrasound Contrast Agents

One approach to make blood easier to detect with ultrasound is to introduce scatterers into the blood to increase its backscatter. To circulate freely and to pass from the venous to the arterial side of the circulation, these particles must be smaller than the capillaries in the lungs are (about 7–10 μm). While being small enough for the circulatory system, the particles must still be efficient acoustic reflectors. The compressibility of gas enables microbubbles to be such efficient scatterers. Unfortunately, free gas bubbles small enough to pass through capillaries are unstable in the blood and dissolve in a fraction of a second due to the combined effects of surface tension and diffusion. To prevent dissolution, bubbles have been stabilized by encapsulation within a shell, and most use a low-solubility, high-molecular-weight gas, such as a perfluorocarbon. The shell is often coated with a biocompatible surfactant to minimize reaction.

Contrast agents for various uses are available from Bracco Diagnostics, GE/Amersham, and Lantheus. Specific application is approved locally by each country. Please check with your local regulatory source for approved agents/applications.

Microbubble Nonlinearity

In this section, we briefly discuss the nonlinear properties of microbubbles [6]. An acoustic wave generated by an ultrasound system consists of alternating high (positive) and low (negative) pressures at frequencies of 1–15 MHz. When an acoustic wave encounters a microbubble, the wave alternately compresses it with the positive pressure and expands it with the negative pressure. During the expansion phase of oscillation, a gas bubble's radius can increase several times, but during contraction, the radius is limited, as the pressure inside gets very high. This results in an asymmetric nonlinear bubble oscillation, which produces harmonics, or multiples of the transmitted frequency. These harmonics help to differentiate microbubbles from tissue, even when they are stationary.

Microbubble Disruption

Once the shell of a microbubble is disrupted, the gas inside will diffuse into the surrounding fluid. The mechanical index (MI), originally defined to predict the onset of cavitation in fluids, also gives an indication of the likelihood of bubble disruption. The MI is defined as:

$$\text{MI} = p_- \, / \, \sqrt{f} \ \text{ or } \ \text{MI} = p_- \times \sqrt{T}$$

where p_- is the peak negative pressure, f is the ultrasound frequency, and T is the ultrasound period [7]. This formula indicates that the harder you try to expand the bubble (peak negative pressure) and the longer you expand it (period of ultrasound wavelength), the more likely it is to break. This phenomenon is also affected by the properties of the particular microbubble shell. More elastic shells are harder to break, as they stretch during negative pressure, without rupturing. It has been well established that the acoustic power level used during routine examinations destroys most contrast microbubbles [8].

The tissue path through which ultrasound travels varies from patient to patient, so the MI displayed on the screen of a commercial device is approximate at best. The acoustic power is measured under ideal conditions and then derated (adjusted) to account for an average amount of attenuation to be expected at the operating frequency. A very conservative estimate is used since the objective of regulatory bodies is to minimize any potential bioeffects of too-high acoustic power. In transcranial imaging, the attenuation and distortion of the skull are typically greater than in other clinical applications, so the power levels used for transcranial applications usually need to be higher to produce the same acoustic pressure at the location of the microbubbles.

The blood flow in a normal capillary bed is on the order of 1 mm/s, and a typical capillary is about 1 mm long [9]. Thus, if the contrast within a capillary is destroyed, it will take about a second or more to refill the capillary. Given the branching structure of the microvasculature and the thickness of a typical scan plane, as well as the flow rate to the organ, it can take several seconds to replenish the contrast in the scan plane.

During real-time scanning at normal output power levels, the contrast is never given a chance to fill the microvasculature. This was first observed by Porter when he found that triggered imaging allows much better visualization of contrast within the myocardium [10]. Similar techniques have been used to image flow in the parenchyma of abdominal organs [11, 12] and the brain [5, 13]. In recent years, new nonlinear imaging techniques have been developed that are far more sensitive to very small returns from microbubbles, making it possible to image them relatively non-destructively in real time at very low acoustic pressures, even through the intact human skull. Some researchers prefer high-MI, low-frame-rate imaging to penetrate into the contralateral hemisphere.

Doppler-Based Techniques

The original intended application of UCAs was to enhance the returned signal from blood and to salvage otherwise failed Doppler exams [14]. This application has not been widely pursued in applications outside neurology due to artifacts seen on ultrasound systems not optimized for the dramatic increase in the signal level provided by the agents [15]. In addition, the sensitivity of ultrasound systems has increased substantially, making this application less important. In transcranial applications, however, some patients' temporal windows are impenetrable without a contrast agent due to attenuation by the skull. Many researchers have found that the use of a contrast agent can salvage most otherwise non-diagnostic exams so that a diagnosis may be made for virtually all patients [16].

Ultrasound contrast research has instead shifted away from the goal of rescuing Doppler exams and toward perfusion measurement, which is the focus of most of the imaging modes described below.

Low-Mechanical-Index Imaging

Low-MI scanning is important for two reasons. First, at an MI of about 0.1 or below, most UCAs are not significantly destroyed yet give a good harmonic contrast signal. In transcranial imaging, an MI of 0.2 or less is used to compensate for skull attenuation. The MI in situ is still around 0.1 or less after the attenuation of the transmitted signal caused by the skull.

The second major reason for low-MI scanning is the reduction of the harmonic component in the tissue echoes relative to the bubble echoes. While tissue harmonics have benefited routine diagnostic scanning, the contrast signal must rise above the background 'noise' signal. Because tissue is less nonlinear than bubbles are, it requires a higher MI than contrast microbubbles do for a certain harmonic response. Therefore, at a low MI, the contrast-to-tissue ratio is higher than at a high MI, helping to remove the tissue signal and leave only the contrast.

Nonlinear Imaging Methods

A number of techniques have been developed to distinguish bubbles from tissue, all of which rely on the higher nonlinearity of bubbles compared with tissue. All of these techniques have their advantages and disadvantages for any particular clinical application, depending largely on whether sensitivity or resolution is the driving factor for that application. Due to the attenuation by the skull, sensitivity tends to dominate the clinical requirements for transcranial imaging.

Harmonic Imaging

'Conventional' harmonic imaging (HI) relies on transmitting at the fundamental frequency f_0 and forming an image from the second harmonic component $2f_0$ of the backscattered echoes by the use of filters to remove the fundamental signal. This restricts the bandwidth available for imaging to ensure that the received harmonic signal can be separated from the fundamental signal, limiting sensitivity and resolution.

While it has long been known that tissue does produce nonlinear energy [17], it was assumed that the higher-frequency harmonics would be eliminated by attenuation. However, it was soon found that tissue did produce significant harmonic energy and that the high sensitivity and bandwidth of modern ultrasound equipment could detect it. In fact, the harmonic image produced by tissue alone has beneficial qualities, such as reduced clutter in the image and improved resolution [18]. Therefore, a tissue image is present even in the absence of a contrast agent, so that perfect separation is not achieved.

Pulse Inversion Imaging

Pulse inversion (PI) imaging avoids the bandwidth limitations of HI by subtracting, rather than filtering out, the fundamental signal [19]. Thus, PI can separate the fundamental component of the bubble echoes from the harmonic, even when they overlap. This allows the use of broader transmit and receive bandwidths for improved resolution and increased sensitivity to contrast agents.

In PI HI, two pulses are transmitted down each ray line. The second pulse is an inverted replica of the first, so that wherever there is positive pressure on the first pulse, there is equal negative pressure on the second. Any linear target that responds equally to positive and negative pressures will reflect back to the transducer, with equal but opposite echoes. These are then added, and all stationary linear targets cancel, as shown in figure 1. Microbubbles respond differently to positive and negative pressures and do not reflect identical inverted waveforms, having both fundamental and harmonic components. Their fundamental components cancel, but their harmonic components add, enhancing the harmonic detection, as also shown in figure 1.

Power Modulation Imaging

An alternative to changing the phase of each successive transmit pulse is to change the amplitude of successive pulses in a group. This technique is referred to as power modulation (PM) imaging. In PM, a low-amplitude transmitted pulse is followed by a higher-amplitude pulse. Upon reception, the lower-amplitude signal is rescaled by the

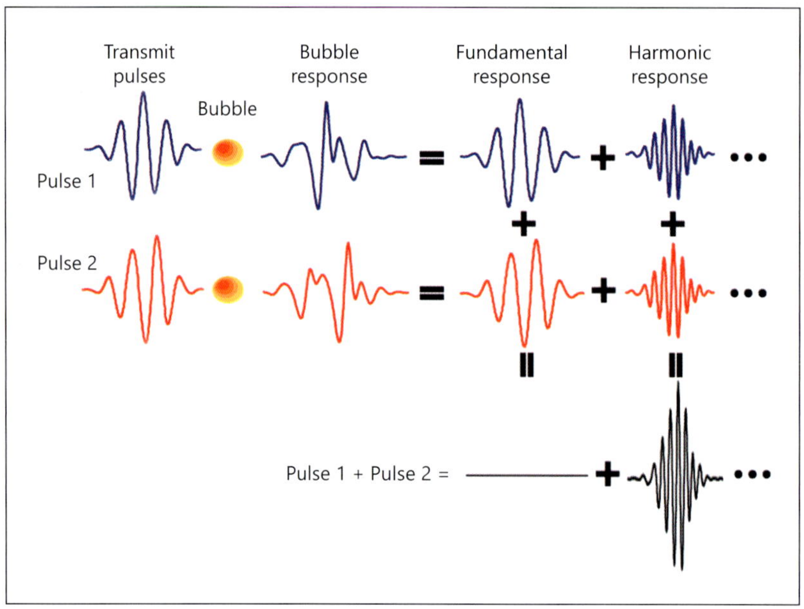

Fig. 1. By adding two consecutive bubble echoes from inverted pulses, pulse inversion cancels fundamental echoes without filtering.

factor between transmit pulses and subtracted. The resulting difference at the fundamental frequency represents energy that has 'leaked out' of the second pulse into the higher harmonics. Figure 2 illustrates the presence of nonlinear fundamental energy in the resulting subtracted spectrum. This lower-frequency nonlinear signal has lower attenuation upon return to the transducer relative to second-harmonic imaging approaches. The increased sensitivity of PM compared with PI makes it ideal for transcranial imaging. For a more detailed comparison of these and other nonlinear imaging methods, see Averkiou et al. [20].

Coded Contrast Harmonics

One of the primary limitations of low-MI contrast imaging is the very low signal levels returned from bubbles at such low acoustic pressures. Tissue imaging typically transmits with 150–200 V, while low-MI contrast imaging uses only 5–10 V. Transmitting any higher voltage will destroy the bubbles. The sensitivity could be increased by transmitting longer pulses, but the axial resolution would suffer. Coded contrast harmonics offer a solution to this apparent dilemma.

Pulse compression is a technique that has been used in radar for decades but that has seen relatively little use in ultrasound. In the case of radar, pulse compression allows transmission of more power without exceeding the voltage limit on the

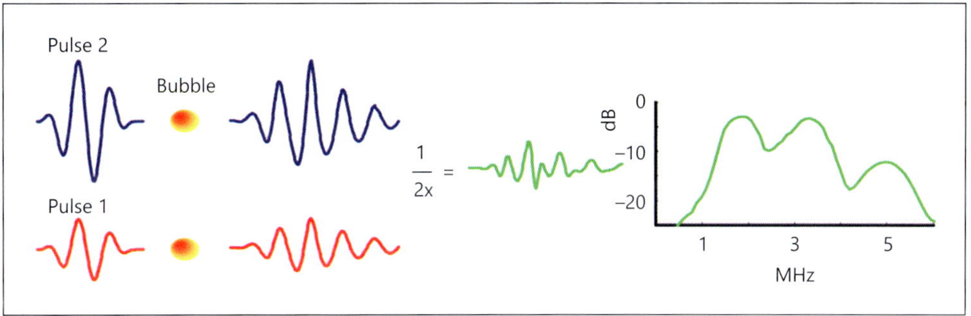

Fig. 2. Power modulation signal processing.

antenna. The basic concept is to transmit a long coded signal that can be compressed back into a short received signal by a filter that has the inverse code of what was transmitted [21]. This allows the voltage to be kept low to avoid bubble destruction but more power to be transmitted since the bursts can be much longer.

A chirp is a commonly used code whose frequency increases over the length of the burst. When correlated with the chirp-decoding filter on reception, the long pulse is compressed back into a short one, as shown in figure 3. This can lead to greater sensitivity with less bubble destruction. Pulse compression methods may be combined with the nonlinear bubble imaging techniques discussed above for highly sensitive contrast imaging, as shown in figure 4a.

Microvascular Imaging

One of the unique aspects of ultrasound contrast imaging is that individual 1–5 μm microbubbles can be easily visualized, even through the skull. Contrast agents used for MR or CT are fluid, so they mix completely with the blood, causing diffuse parenchymal enhancement in tissue. The ability to visualize individual microbubbles in real time allows one to see them in small vessels (<1 mm) in regions with very low blood flow velocities (<1 cm/s). In some vessels, the flow rate is so low that a bubble may pass through only every few seconds. It might be visible for several frames but still gives only a fleeting glimpse of the vasculature.

Microvascular imaging (MVI) tracks the passage of microbubbles through these smaller vessels. This processing measures changes in the image from frame to frame, suppressing any background tissue signal, capturing the bubbles as they pass through. This enhances vessel conspicuity, showing the tracks of single bubbles flowing through the microvasculature, as shown in figure 4b. To capture the images in figure 4, a normal bolus of contrast was injected to capture the perfusion image in figure 4a. Then, after the bolus faded, MVI was enabled to capture the vasculature shown in figure 4b from the tracks of the remaining bubbles.

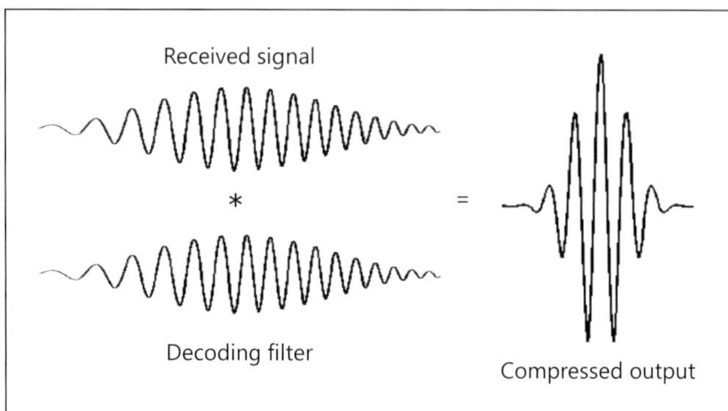

Fig. 3. Pulse compression showing the received signal, the decoding filter, and the compressed output.

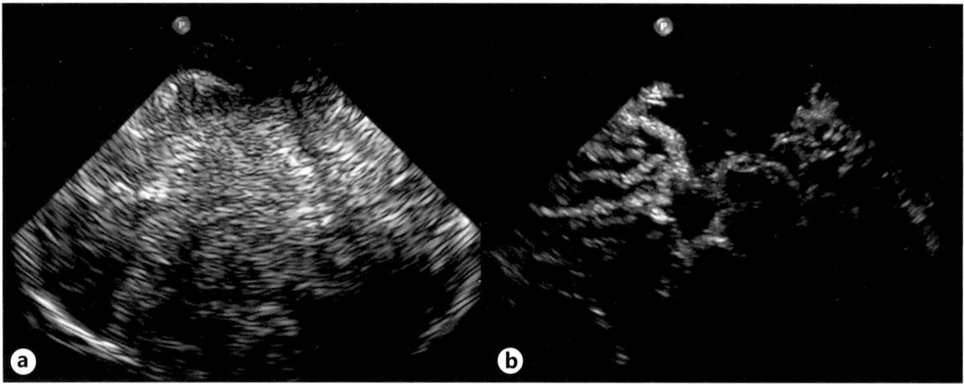

Fig. 4. Perfusion and vascular contrast imaging. **a** Perfusion image at the peak of bolus injection; **b** MVI image after integrating the tracks of many bubbles over several seconds.

Flash Contrast Imaging

While the ability to visualize microvascular blood flow in real time is a significant advancement, the ability to disrupt contrast is also useful. The techniques described above can detect nearly stationary microbubbles in the microcirculation. Flash contrast imaging enables visualization of the arterial vasculature of a lesion after the microcirculation fills. Flash refers to the transmission of a few high-MI frames to clear a plane of contrast agent, followed by a return to low-MI imaging.

When an intravenous bolus of contrast first arrives in the arterial vessels, it provides visualization of the arterial vasculature. However, once the microcirculation fills with microbubbles, the larger arterial vasculature is obscured, as seen in figure 4a. Flash contrast imaging is often employed with MVI to see vascular flow while the bolus is still near its peak. Flash contrast imaging also holds promise as a quantification technique by creating a localized negative bolus of contrast and then measuring the refill kinetics. This use is described below in the 'Contrast Quantification Techniques' section.

Contrast Quantification Techniques

Contrast ultrasound provides opportunities for quantification that may lead to improved diagnosis, therapy monitoring, and patient prognosis. Substantial literature exists on indicator dilution techniques using a contrast bolus [22, 23]. Volumetric blood flow measurement with contrast ultrasound using indicator dilution techniques is not yet possible due to the requirement of knowing the absolute concentration of the agent. However, measurements of bolus kinetics, such as the arrival time, time to peak, or time to wash-out, do hold promise for diagnosing several disease states in general radiology [24, 25]. The ability to image perfusion with UCAs is showing promise for differentiating ischemic from normal brain tissue [26].

Flash contrast imaging also holds promise for flow quantification. Contrast enhancement in an image actually represents the volume of contrast within the image, and not the flow rate. The flow rate is more closely related to perfusion than the blood volume is; the blood volume in the brain is highly autoregulated and nearly constant, even in regions of widely varying flow rates. If a stenosis restricts the blood flow entering a volume of tissue, it will be slow to fill with contrast, but once the vascular bed has filled with contrast, it may be difficult to differentiate the reduced flow rate.

Contrast within a scan plane can be cleared using a 'flash pulse' (see the 'Flash Contrast Imaging' section), creating a 'negative bolus' of contrast locally. The time that it takes for the contrast to refill the scan plane is an indicator of the local blood flow velocity. This has been proposed as a method for the quantification of myocardial perfusion [27, 28] and for neurological applications, such as stroke detection or penumbra definition [26]. Contrast infusion is often used to provide a stable contrast concentration over the duration of the exam.

Research is underway on the clinical applications of ultrasound contrast imaging in the field of neurology. As contrast imaging techniques improve and as research to reduce or mitigate aberrations and attenuation by the skull continues, even more clinical uses of UCAs are likely to be developed.

References

1 Feinstein SB, Cheirif J, Ten CF, Silverman PR, Heidenreich PA, Dick C, et al: Safety and efficacy of a new transpulmonary ultrasound contrast agent: initial multicenter clinical results. J Am Coll Cardiol 1990;16:316–324.

2 Schneider M: Characteristics of SonoVue (TM). Echocardiography 1999;16:743–746.

3 Burns PN, Powers JE, Hope Simpson D, Uhlendorf V, Fritzsch T: Harmonic imaging: principles and preliminary results. Angiology 1996;47:S63–S74.

4 Claassen L, Seidel G, Algermissen C: Quantification of flow rates using harmonic grey-scale imaging and an ultrasound contrast agent: an in vitro and in vivo study. Ultrasound Med Biol 2001;27:83–88.

5 Wiesmann M, Seidel G: Ultrasound perfusion imaging of the human brain. Stroke 2000;31:2421–2425.

6 Leighton TG: The Acoustic Bubble. London, UK, Academic Press, 1994.

7 Apfel RE, Holland CK: Gauging the likelihood of cavitation from short-pulse, low-duty cycle diagnostic ultrasound. Ultrasound Med Biol 1991;17:179–185.

8 Villarraga HR, Foley DA, Aeschbacher BC, Klarich KW, Mulvagh SL: Destruction of contrast microbubbles during ultrasound imaging at conventional power output. J Am Soc Echocardiography 1997;10: 783–791.

9 Berne RM, Levy MN: Cardiovascular Physiology, ed 2. St. Louis, C.V. Mosby Co., 1972, p 265.

10 Porter TR, Xie F: Transient myocardial contrast after initial exposure to diagnostic ultrasound pressures with minute doses of intravenously injected microbubbles. Demonstration and potential mechanisms. Circulation 1995;92:2391–2395.

11 Heckemann RA, Cosgrove DO, Blomley MJ, Eckersley RJ, Harvey CJ, Mine Y: Liver lesions: intermittent second-harmonic gray-scale US can increase conspicuity with microbubble contrast material-early experience. Radiology 2000;216:592–596.

12 Wilson SR, Burns PN, Muradali D, Wilson JA, Lai X: Harmonic hepatic US with microbubble contrast agent: initial experience showing improved characterization of hemangioma, hepatocellular carcinoma, and metastasis. Radiology 2000;215:153–161.

13 Seidel G, Meyer K: Harmonic imaging – a new method for the sonographic assessment of cerebral perfusion. Eur J Ultrasound 2001;14:103–113.

14 Burns PN, Hilpert P, Goldberg BB: Intravenous contrast agent for ultrasound Doppler: in vivo measurement of small vessel dose-response. Proc Twelfth Ann Int Conf IEEE Eng Med Biol Soc, 1990, pp 322–324.

15 Forsberg F, Liu JB, Burns PN, Merton DA, Goldberg BB: Artifacts in ultrasonic contrast agent studies. J Ultrasound Med 1994;13:357–365.

16 Seidel G, Meairs S: Ultrasound contrast agents in ischemic stroke. Cerebrovasc Dis 2009;27(suppl 2):25–39.

17 Hamiltion MF, Blackstock DT: Nonlinear Acoustics. San Diego, CA, Academic Press, 1998.

18 Averkiou MA, Roundhill DN, Powers JE: New imaging technique based on the nonlinear properties of tissues. Proc IEEE Ultrasonics Symposium, Toronto, Ontario, 1997, pp 1561–1566.

19 Burns PN, Wilson SR, Simpson DH: Pulse inversion imaging of liver blood flow: improved method for characterizing focal masses with microbubble contrast. Invest Radiol 2000;35:58–71.

20 Averkiou M, Mannaris C, Bruce M, Powers J: Nonlinear pulsing schemes for the detection of ultrasound contrast agents. 155th Meeting of the Acoustical Society of America, Paris, 2008, pp 915–920.

21 Borsboom JM, Chin CT, de Jong N: Nonlinear coded excitation method for ultrasound contrast imaging. Ultrasound Med Biol 2003;29:277–284.

22 Bassingthwaighte J: Physiology and theory of tracer washout techniques for the estimation of myocardial blood flow: flow estimation from tracer washout. Prog Cardiovasc Dis 1977;20:165–189.

23 Blomley MJ, Dawson P: Bolus dynamics: theoretical and experimental aspects. Br J Radiol 1997;70:351–359.

24 Albrecht T, Blomley MJ, Cosgrove DO, Taylor-Robinson SD, Jayaram V, Eckersley R, et al: Non-invasive diagnosis of hepatic cirrhosis by transit-time analysis of an ultrasound contrast agent. Lancet 1999;353:1579–1583.

25 Blomley MJ, Lim AK, Harvey CJ, Patel N, Eckersley RJ, Basilico R, et al: Liver microbubble transit time compared with histology and Child-Pugh score in diffuse liver disease: a cross sectional study. Gut 2003;52:1188–1193.

26 Kern R, Diels A, Pettenpohl J, Kablau M, Brade J, Hennerici MG, et al: Real-time ultrasound brain perfusion imaging with analysis of microbubble replenishment in acute MCA stroke. J Cereb Blood Flow Metab 2011;31:1716–1724.

27 Averkiou M, Bruce M, Powers J (inventors); ATL Ultrasound (assignee): Ultrasonic diagnostic imaging with contrast agents. USA patent 5,833,613. 1998.

28 Wei K, Jayaweera AR, Firoozan S, Linka A, Skyba DM, Kaul S: Quantification of myocardial blood flow with ultrasound-induced destruction of microbubbles administered as a constant venous infusion. Circulation 1998;97:473–483.

Jeff Powers, PhD
Principal Scientist
Philips Ultrasound, MS1010
22100 Bothell Hwy
Bothell, WA 98021 (USA)
E-Mail jeff.powers@philips.com

Alonso A, Hennerici MG, Meairs S (eds): Translational Neurosonology.
Front Neurol Neurosci. Basel, Karger, 2015, vol 36, pp 11–22 (DOI: 10.1159/000366223)

Physical Principles of Microbubbles for Ultrasound Imaging and Therapy

Eleanor Stride

Department of Mechanical Engineering, University College London, London, UK

Abstract

Microbubble ultrasound contrast agents have been in clinical use for more than two decades, during which time their range of applications has increased to encompass echocardiography, Doppler enhancement, perfusion studies and molecular imaging, as well as a number of therapeutic applications, including drug delivery, gene therapy, high-intensity focused ultrasound treatments and sonothrombolysis. The aim of this article is to review the different types of microbubble agents, their physical behaviours and the mechanisms underlying their effectiveness in imaging and therapeutic applications.   © 2015 S. Karger AG, Basel

Introduction

Microbubbles have now been in clinical use as contrast agents for ultrasound imaging for more than two decades. Their primary application is currently in echocardiography for ventricular opacification and the delineation of endocardial borders [1], although they have also been used successfully for the assessment of systolic function and left ventricular volume [2] and for identifying myocardial infarction and coronary artery stenosis [3]. The development of harmonic imaging, together with advances in three-dimensional visualisation techniques, have further enabled the mapping of microcirculation using microbubbles, for example, in the characterisation of tumour vascularity [4] and also in the brain, offering substantial advantages in the assessment of stroke patients [5]. Other non-vascular applications of microbubbles include the assessment of fallopian tube patency [6] and the detection of ureteric reflux [7].

Microbubbles have also shown great potential in quantitative and targeted (molecular) imaging. In addition to providing a means of signal enhancement in Doppler studies [8], they enable the measurement of parameters such as relative vascular volume, flow velocity and perfusion rate. This has been demonstrated in a number of applications, including the diagnosis and treatment monitoring of liver tumours [9] and the assessment of myocardial function [3]. There are still some significant challenges to be overcome before fully quantitative imaging protocols can be developed [10], but they are being actively pursued. The ability to attach molecules to microbubbles that are targeted to specific vascular receptor sites has opened up further opportunities for molecular imaging, and conditions currently under investigation include inflammation, angiogenesis and atherosclerosis [11].

Another area that has been the subject of intensive research is the use of microbubbles in therapeutic applications. In high intensity-focused ultrasound surgery, microbubbles have been used as a means of nucleating the cavitation in the target volume to increase the speed and efficacy of the treatment [12]. In drug delivery and gene therapy, microbubbles can be used as vehicles that are loaded with the required therapeutic agent, traced to the target site using low-intensity ultrasound and then destroyed with a high-intensity burst to release the material locally, thus avoiding systemic administration, e.g. for toxic chemotherapy [13]. Moreover, there is considerable evidence that the motion of the microbubbles increases the permeability of both individual cell membranes and the endothelium, including the temporary opening of the blood-brain barrier [14]. Perhaps one of the most exciting therapeutic applications of microbubbles is in sonothrombolysis, for which they have been shown to markedly increase the effectiveness of tissue plasminogen activator and the rate of clot lysis in vitro and in vivo [15]. The aim of this chapter is to provide an overview of the physical behaviours of microbubbles and the mechanisms underlying their effectiveness in imaging and therapeutic applications.

Basic Physics of Microbubbles

Stability

An uncoated gas microbubble is subject to very high interfacial (surface) tension at the boundary between the gas and the surrounding liquid. This can be represented as excess pressure acting on the bubble surface:

$$\Delta p = \frac{2\sigma}{R}$$

where Δp is the excess pressure (normally known as the Laplace Pressure), σ is the interfacial tension and R is the bubble radius. For an air bubble having a diameter of a few microns (i.e. $R < 10^{-5}$ m) in water, Δp will be very high (~0.1 MPa). Hence, there is a need for contrast agent microbubbles with a stabilising coating, which will both reduce interfacial tension and provide a physical barrier to gas diffusion, thus preventing them from dissolving too rapidly (fig. 1).

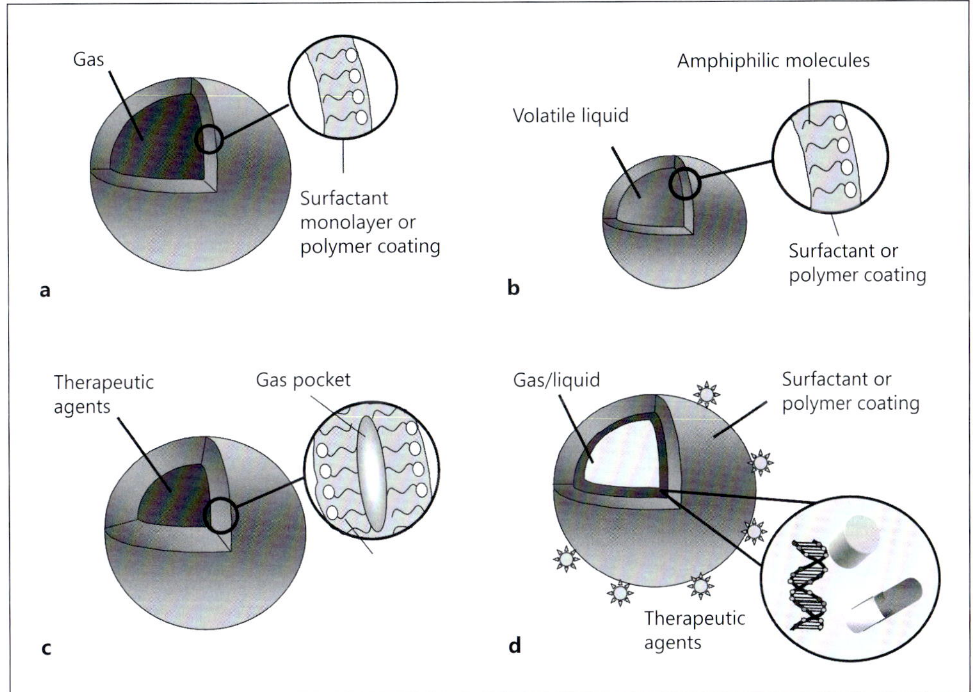

Fig. 1. Different types of microbubble agents used for ultrasound imaging and therapy: (**a**) coated microbubble, (**b**) phase-shift emulsion, (**c**) echogenic liposome, (**d**) multi-layered microbubble.

Response to Ultrasound

Because they are filled with gas, microbubbles are highly compressible, and when they are exposed to an ultrasound field, the varying pressures cause them to expand and contract (fig. 2). It is these volume oscillations that are the key to the effectiveness of microbubbles both as ultrasound contrast agents and in therapeutic applications, which will be explained in the subsequent sections.

The natures of these oscillations may be classified into four groups, depending upon the frequencies and pressures at which the microbubbles are excited and their resulting amplitudes of oscillation:

(i) Linear Oscillations

At low excitation pressures, the microbubbles exhibit small-amplitude, stable, symmetrical oscillations at the same frequency as the incident field (fig. 2a). The microbubble coating remains intact, and the maximum amplitude of oscillation is observed at the linear resonance frequency.

(ii) Non-Linear Oscillations

As the amplitude of the excitation pressure increases, so does the amplitude of the microbubble oscillations, which then become non-symmetrical, i.e. the microbubble

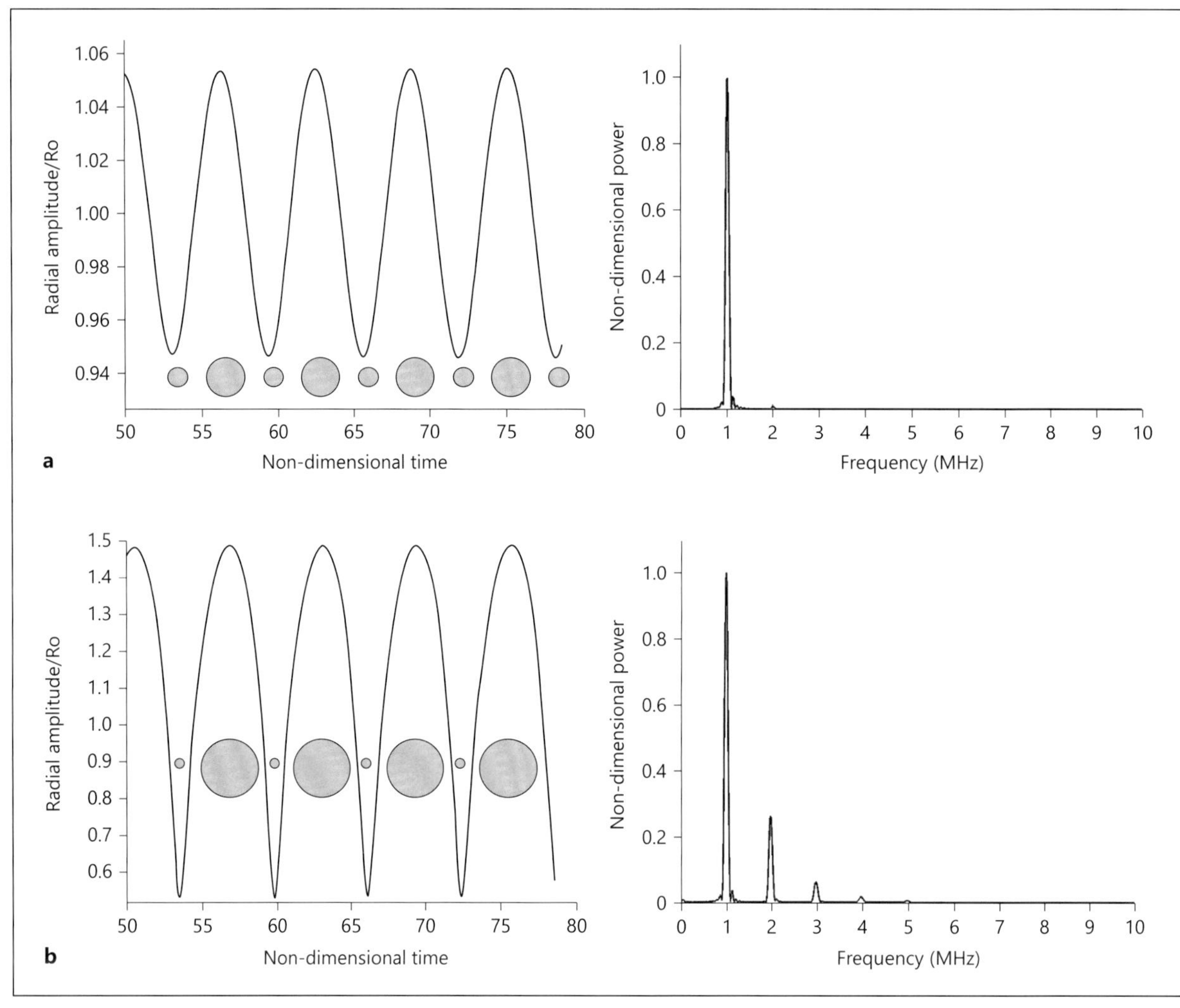

Fig. 2. Characteristics of microbubble oscillation. Plots showing the changes in microbubble radii and the frequency spectra of the radiated ultrasound fields for bubbles undergoing: (**a**) linear oscillations, (**b**) non-linear oscillations, (**c**) stable cavitation, (**d**) inertial cavitation.

may expand to a greater degree than it compresses or vice versa. It may also undergo non-spherical and/or surface oscillations. This non-linear behaviour is reflected by the frequency spectrum of the sound field radiated by the microbubbles, which contain not only the frequency at which they were excited but also the harmonics and sub-/ultraharmonics (i.e. multiples and fractions) of this frequency (fig. 2b).

For this group, the microbubble coating remains intact, at least initially, although it may undergo alterations, leading to bubble shrinkage and/or a gradual change in the amplitude of oscillation. This depends upon the specific coating and may vary from bubble to bubble even within a given population. Similarly, the amplitude at

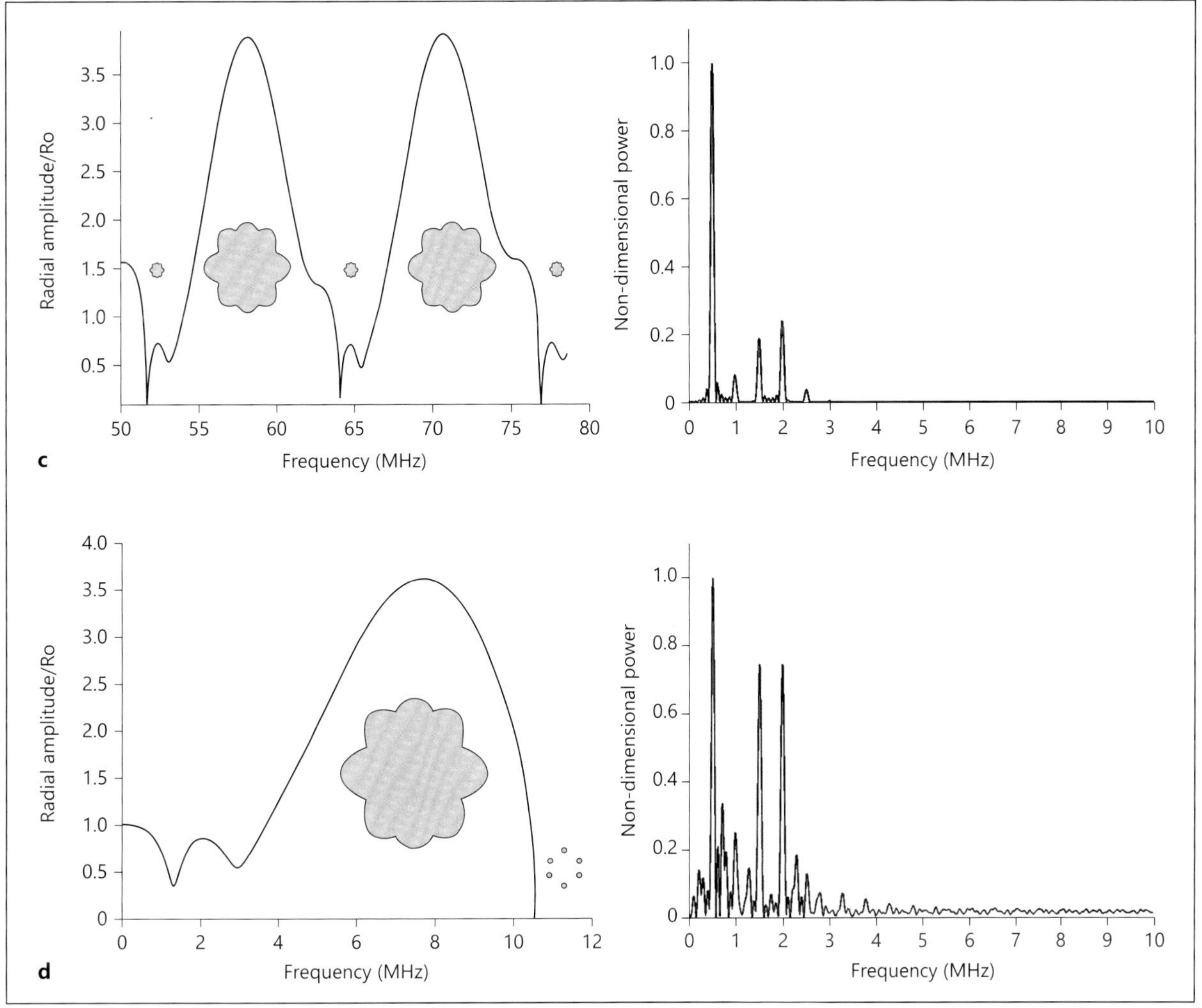

which non-linear effects are observed depends upon the microbubble coating. Some phospholipid-coated bubbles exhibit non-linear behaviours at very low amplitudes [16], whilst some polymer-coated bubbles exhibit almost entirely linear behaviours up to relatively high pressures.

Consequently, predicting microbubble behaviours theoretically under these conditions becomes increasingly complex. Moreover, the frequency at which the amplitude of oscillation is maximised becomes pressure dependent and can no longer be predicted by a simple equation, and the interactions of the microbubbles both with their surroundings and each other becomes increasingly important [17, 18].

(iii) Stable Cavitation

Beyond a certain excitation pressure, the response of the microbubble is no longer significantly affected by the coating, and it behaves effectively as an uncoated gas bubble, undergoing stable (i.e. repetitive) but highly non-linear oscillations controlled by the balance between the pressure of the gas inside the bubble and the inertia of the surrounding liquid. Hence, the frequency spectrum of the radiated sound field then contains a substantial harmonic content due to both volume oscillations and surface oscillations, which are more likely in the absence of the constraint caused by the coating (fig. 2c).

(iv) Inertial Cavitation

At even higher pressures, the bubble is able to grow so large during the expansion phase that the internal pressure becomes too low to support the inertia of the surrounding liquid, and the bubble collapses inwards upon itself very rapidly [19]. This is an extremely violent process, the effects of which will be discussed subsequently, and it normally results in the bubble breaking up into small fragments. Depending upon the amplitude, frequency, pulse repetition frequency and duty cycle of the ultrasound field, these fragments may either dissolve away (under surface tension) or undergo rectified diffusion and grow to form new bubbles, which eventually undergo the same process. Similarly, under the right conditions, a bubble initially undergoing stable cavitation may grow to a sufficient size for inertial collapse to occur. Once inertial cavitation has started, the radiated sound field will no longer contain discrete harmonic components but rather broadband noise (i.e. the energy is distributed continuously across a wide range of frequencies) (fig. 2d).

Mechanisms of Image Contrast Enhancement

There are a number of reasons why microbubbles are so effective as ultrasound contrast agents:

Impedance Contrast
First, the high compressibility of gas microbubbles compared with that of their surroundings gives rise to a large difference in acoustic impedance between the microbubbles and the liquid in which they are suspended. Thus, there will be a strong reflection from any region containing microbubbles as there would be from any region in the body containing gas (e.g. lung, bowel).

Resonant Reradiation
Second, the fact that the microbubbles undergo volume oscillations means that they not only reflect but also absorb and re-radiate sound energy to a much greater extent than liquid-filled particles of similar sizes, such as red blood cells (i.e. their echogenicity would still be considerably higher even if the impedance contrast with the sur-

rounding liquid were the same for both the microbubbles and blood cells). There is, moreover, a fortuitous coincidence between the size of the microbubble able to pass through human capillaries (<8 μm) and that which is resonant at the frequencies typically used for ultrasound imaging (1–15 MHz). Thus, the amplitudes of the microbubble oscillations, and hence, the contrast enhancing effects, are maximised under diagnostic conditions.

Non-Linear Response
It is, however, the non-linear characteristic of the microbubble oscillations that is perhaps the most important factor in terms of image contrast enhancement. As described above, if microbubbles are excited at a sufficient amplitude, the re-radiated sound field will contain distinct harmonics (whole and fractional) of the excitation frequency. This enables the microbubble signal to be distinguished from that produced by the surrounding tissue, which will contain a much smaller proportion of the harmonics. The ultrasound system can be tuned to receive at a particular harmonic and to use this information for creating the image [20]. Because the harmonic components will be due predominantly to the microbubbles rather than to the surrounding tissue, the signal:noise (or bubble:tissue) ratio can be greatly increased. The second harmonic is the most commonly used frequency component, but the possibilities of using higher harmonics, subharmonics and ultraharmonics of the insonation frequency have also been investigated [21].

This type of direct harmonic imaging has two main disadvantages. First, image resolution is limited because the bandwidth of the transmitting transducer must be kept narrow to avoid overlap between the fundamental and second harmonic in the received signal. Second, whilst it is true that the harmonic content of the received signal is due mainly to the microbubbles, the contribution from the surrounding tissue is not entirely negligible at the pressures required to promote significantly non-linear microbubble behaviours. Alternative imaging strategies have been devised to overcome these drawbacks. For example, in 'pulse inversion imaging' [22], an initial imaging pulse is transmitted and followed, after a suitable delay, by an inverted copy of itself. If the two pulses are scattered linearly, the sum of the resulting echoes will be zero. If, however, they encounter non-linear scatterers, such as microbubbles, there will be a residual signal after summation, which will be proportional to the degree of non-linearity (fig. 3). Using this signal for image generation enables superior image resolution to be attained because in this case, the signal bandwidth does not need to be limited. The principle of pulse inversion has formed the basis for a wide range of novel imaging strategies, including amplitude and phase-modulation imaging [23].

Destruction
A further feature of microbubble behaviours that can be exploited for imaging is the fact that they can be rapidly destroyed by increasing the amplitude of excitation. This results not only in a strongly non-linear signal being produced during the destruction

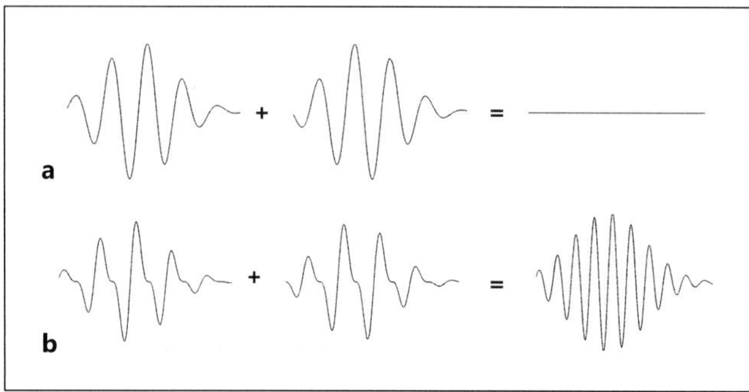

Fig. 3. Principle of pulse inversion imaging. Two pulses are transmitted, which are separated by a short delay, and the second pulse is an inverted copy of the first: (**a**) if the two pulses are linearly propagated, then summing them will produce a zero signal; (**b**) if they are non-linearly propagated, then their sum will produce a finite signal.

process itself due to the unencapsulated gas bubbles produced but also in a distinct change in the nature of the signal before and after the destruction has taken place. This registers as a strong transient signal in the Doppler imaging mode and enables the sensitivity for detecting small features, such as metastases, to be greatly increased [24].

Microbubble Phenomena in Therapeutic Applications: Physical Effects

In addition to having significant effects upon the sound field, oscillating microbubbles can also produce a range of physical phenomena, the effects of which may be beneficial or harmful depending on the location of the microbubbles and the type of oscillations. Further discussion of the safety of microbubbles may be found in reference [25].

Primary Radiation Force
A propagating ultrasound wave has associated momentum, which can be transferred to objects located in the beam path. The resultant force experienced by the object is known as the primary radiation or Bjerknes force, and if the object is free to move, it will undergo translation in the direction of the beam. It has been suggested that this effect could be exploited as a means of targeting microbubbles by driving them into the target region. Merely pushing the bubbles against the cell repetitively may be sufficient to stimulate cell uptake [26]. At high ultrasound pressures, bubbles have been shown to translate very rapidly in vitro (5–10 cm/s) and to be capable of destroying cells upon impact. However, in vivo, this 'bubble bullet' effect does not appear to be significant, possibly because a very high bubble:cell ratio is required or because the presence of carbon dioxide in the blood has a damping effect on bubble activity.

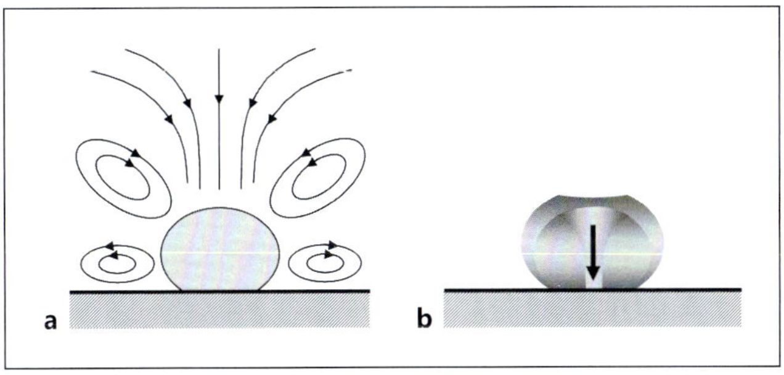

Fig. 4. Physical phenomena relevant to microbubble-mediated ultrasound therapy: (**a**) microstreaming and (**b**) microjet formation near a surface.

Secondary Radiation Force

Oscillating microbubbles act as secondary sources of sound, so they also have a radiation force associated with them. This secondary radiation (Bjerknes) force may cause attraction between the microbubbles and nearby particles (e.g. blood cells) and between the microbubbles themselves [27]. It may also cause a microbubble to become attached to a nearby surface that is reflecting the radiated sound. This may have a direct effect if the pulsation of the bubble is of a sufficient amplitude to damage the cell (although attachment may affect the bubble's ability to pulsate). The increased proximity may also contribute to the effects produced by microstreaming and microjetting (see below).

Microstreaming

The absorption of energy from the propagating wave by the surrounding fluid causes a transfer of momentum that sets up a steady current or 'streaming' in the direction of the beam (fig. 4a). Similar effects are observed on a smaller scale around microbubbles undergoing stable oscillations, which on account of their spherical geometries, manifest as eddying motions. These flows may, in turn, impose shear stresses on nearby surfaces, such as cell membranes, and it has been suggested that this may be the cause of the stimulated uptake observed upon the exposure of cells to ultrasound in the presence of microbubbles. At higher amplitudes of microbubble oscillation and, hence, higher shear stresses, microstreaming has been shown to cause significant damage to cells [28], and it is also thought to be responsible for the eroding effects observed in sonothrombolysis. The fact that the rate of clot dissolution was found to be enhanced more by stable than by inertial cavitation (which does not generate significant microstreaming) supports this hypothesis [29]. Microstreaming also contributes to the circulation of therapeutic agents in the target region, which is likely to be important in the context of sonothrombolysis and tissue plasminogen activator uptake.

Microjetting

If a microbubble undergoes inertial collapse close to a rigid surface, the asymmetry in the motion of the liquid may cause the bubble to 'turn in' upon itself (fig. 4b), producing a high-speed micro-jet travelling towards the surface. The impact of this jet may be sufficient to puncture a cell membrane, and this effect has been observed extensively in vitro, including with contrast agents near cells [30]. It has been suggested that this could also be the cause of the enhanced cell uptake generated by microbubbles, but on account of the relatively high ultrasound pressures required and the consequent risk of permanent cell damage, it is more generally thought that stable cavitation phenomena, such as microstreaming, are more likely to be associated with reversible sonoporation.

Inertial Collapse
As described above, at high amplitudes of excitation, microbubbles may collapse violently, releasing energy in the form of a shock wave, which may directly damage the surrounding tissue. The heating and chemical effects associated with inertial cavitation are discussed below.

Thermal Effects

In addition to promoting streaming, the absorption of energy that occurs as ultrasound waves propagate through a medium produces a heating effect. In most materials, including tissues, the rate of absorption increases with frequency, and thus, the presence of bubbles can enhance this heating effect due to their abilities to generate higher harmonics of the excitation frequency. Bubbles will also dissipate energy as heat as a result of viscous friction in the surrounding liquid and coating material and via conduction during compression. The relative significance of each of these dissipation mechanisms depends upon the size of the bubble, the physical properties of the surrounding liquid and the frequency and intensity of the ultrasound field. Similarly, the magnitude of the temperature rise generated will also depend upon these parameters as well as the concentration of bubbles present, the pulse repetition frequency/duty cycle and the proximity to blood vessels. Large temperature rises are clearly beneficial for tissue ablation, e.g. for high-intensity focused ultrasound surgery and for certain types of drug and gene delivery systems in which thermal activation is required. For diagnostic imaging and for therapeutic agents that are temperature sensitive, however, significant heating is normally undesirable, and the relevance of safety indices (e.g. thermal index) for applications employing microbubbles requires further investigation.

It is worth briefly discussing the temperature rise occurring inside of a bubble undergoing inertial collapse. By definition, this process involves a very large and rapid reduction in volume and, consequently, a significant rise in pressure and temperature (several thousand kelvins or more). However, these extreme conditions are confined to the centre of the bubble because the bubble will start to expand before the energy can be transferred to the surroundings (with the rate of heat transfer being much lower than the frequency at which the bubble is oscillating). Hilgenfeldt et al. have shown that the temperature rise in the liquid at just a few micrometres from the bubble centre should be relatively negligible (<1 K) and persist for no more than a few microseconds.

Chemical Effects

It is well known that the high temperatures and pressures generated at the centre of a bubble as a result of inertial cavitation collapse may produce highly reactive chemical species, which is a phenomenon that is utilised extensively in chemical engineering. Of particular interest in the context of medical ultrasound is the potential for the formation of free radicals and toxic chemicals, such as hydrogen peroxide (H_2O_2). Their significance has been implicated in observations of cell damage away from the site of direct ultrasound exposure, and high concentrations of these species have been reported in the presence of contrast agent microbubbles [31].

Perhaps more important, particularly for therapeutic applications, are the chemical reactions occurring at the cell membrane during low-intensity ultrasound exposure in the presence of microbubbles. This is an area that has only recently started to be investigated in detail. For example, Juffermans et al. have shown that rat cardiomyoblast cells experience a calcium ion (Ca^{2+}) influx upon exposure to low-intensity ultrasound with SonoVue® [32], causing the localised hyperpolarisation of the cell membrane, which may promote molecular uptake. The underlying cause of this effect is still unclear, although it may also be related to the generation of H_2O_2, despite the much lower ultrasound intensities. Due to the lack of current detailed studies, future developments will be of great importance in optimising the use of microbubbles in therapeutic procedures and in the assessment of their safety for use in both imaging and therapy.

References

1 Al-Mansour HA, Mulvagh SL, Pumper GM, et al: Usefulness of harmonic imaging for left ventricular opacification and endocardial border delineation by optison. Am J Cardiol 2000;85:795–799, A10.

2 Porter TR, Xie F, Kricsfeld A: The mechanism and clinical implication of improved left ventricular videointensity following intravenous injection of multifold dilutions of albumin with dextrose. Int J Card Imaging 1995;11:117–125.

3 Lindner JR, Wei K, Kaul S: Imaging of myocardial perfusion with sonovue (TM) in patients with a prior myocardial infarction. Echocardiography 1999;16: 753–760.

4 McDonald DM, Choyke PL: Imaging of angiogenesis: from microscope to clinic. Nat Med 2003;9:713–725.

5 Meairs S: Contrast-enhanced ultrasound perfusion imaging in acute stroke patients. Eur Neurol 2008;59: 17–26.

6 Prefumo F, Serafini G, Martinoli C, et al: The sonographic evaluation of tubal patency with stimulated acoustic emission imaging. Ultrasound Obstet Gynecol 2002;20:386–389.

7 Darge K, Moeller RT, Trusen A, et al: Diagnosis of vesicoureteric reflux with low-dose contrast-enhanced harmonic ultrasound imaging. Pediatr Radiol 2005;35:73–78.

8 Bleeker H, Shung K, Barnhart J: On the application of ultrasonic contrast agents for blood flowmetry and assessment of cardiac perfusion. J Ultrasound Med 1990;9:461–471.

9 Leen E, Ceccotti P, Kalogeropoulou C, et al: Prospective multicenter trial evaluating a novel method of characterizing focal liver lesions using contrast-enhanced sonography. AJR Am J Roentgenol 2006; 186:1551–1559.

10 Tang MX, Mulvana H, Gauthier T, et al: Quantitative contrast-enhanced ultrasound imaging: a review of sources of variability. Interface Focus 2011;1:520–539.

11 Kaufmann BA, Lindner JR: Molecular imaging with targeted contrast ultrasound. Curr Opin Biotechnol 2007;18:11–16.

12 Luo W, Zhou XD, Ren XL, et al: Enhancing effects of sonovue, a microbubble sonographic contrast agent, on high-intensity focused ultrasound ablation in rabbit livers in vivo. J Ultrasound Med 2007;26:469–476.

13 Bull JL: The application of microbubbles for targeted drug delivery. Expert Opin Drug Deliv 2007;4:475–493.

14 Meairs S, Alonso A: Ultrasound, microbubbles and the blood-brain barrier. Prog Biophys Mol Biol 2007; 93:354–362.

15 Molina CA, Ribo M, Rubiera M, et al: Microbubble administration accelerates clot lysis during continuous 2-mHz ultrasound monitoring in stroke patients treated with intravenous tissue plasminogen activator. Stroke 2006;37:425–429.

16 De Jong N, Emmer M, Chin CT, et al: 'Compression-only' behavior of phospholipid-coated contrast bubbles. Ultrasound Med Biol 2007;33:653–656.

17 Stride E, Saffari N: Investigating the significance of multiple scattering in ultrasound contrast agent particle populations. IEEE Trans Ultrason Ferroelectr Freq Control 2005;52:2332–2345.

18 Qin SP, Ferrara KW: Acoustic response of compliable microvessels containing ultrasound contrast agents. Phys Med Biol 2006;51:5065–5088.

19 Flynn HG: Physics of acoustic cavitation. J Acoust Soc Am 1959;31:1582–1582.

20 Schrope B, Newhouse VL, Uhlendorf V: Simulated capillary blood-flow measurement using a nonlinear ultrasonic contrast agent. Ultrason Imaging 1992; 14:134–158.

21 Forsberg F, Shi WT, Goldberg BB: Subharmonic imaging of contrast agents. Ultrasonics 2000;38:93–98.

22 Krishnan S, O'Donnell M: Transmit aperture processing for nonlinear contrast agent imaging. Ultrason Imaging 1996;18:77–105.

23 Eckersley RJ, Chin CT, Burns PN: Optimising phase and amplitude modulation schemes for imaging microbubble contrast agents at low acoustic power. Ultrasound Med Biol 2005;31:213–219.

24 Harvey CJ, Blomley MJK, Eckersley RJ, et al: Pulse-inversion mode imaging of liver specific microbubbles: improved detection of subcentimetre metastases. Lancet 2000;355:807–808.

25 Nyborg W: Wfumb safety symposium on echo-contrast agents: mechanisms for the interaction of ultrasound. Ultrasound Med Biol 2007;33:224–232.

26 van Wamel A, Kooiman K, Harteveld M, et al: Vibrating microbubbles poking individual cells: drug transfer into cells via sonoporation. J Control Release 2006;112:149–155.

27 Postema M, Van Wamel A, Lancée CT, et al: Ultrasound-induced encapsulated microbubble phenomena. Ultrasound Med Biol 2004;30:827–840.

28 Marmottant P, Biben T, Hilgenfeldt S: Deformation and rupture of lipid vesicles in the strong shear flow generated by ultrasound-driven microbubbles. P R Soc A 2008;464:1781–1800.

29 Datta S, Coussios CC, McAdory LE, et al: Correlation of cavitation with ultrasound enhancement of thrombolysis. Ultrasound Med Biol 2006;32:1257–1267.

30 Prentice P, Cuschieri A, Dholakia K, et al: Membrane disruption by optically controlled microbubble cavitation. Nat Phys 2005;1:107–110.

31 Riesz P, Kondo T: Free radical formation induced by ultrasound and its biological implications. Free Radic Biol Med 1992;13:247–270.

32 Juffermans LJM, Kamp O, Dijkmans PA, et al: Low-intensity ultrasound-exposed microbubbles provoke local hyperpolarization of the cell membrane via activation of BK(Ca) channels. Ultrasound Med Biol 2008;34:502–508.

Eleanor Stride, PhD
Department of Mechanical Engineering, University College London
Torrington Place
London WC1E 7JE (UK)
E-Mail e_stride@meng.ucl.ac.uk

Alonso A, Hennerici MG, Meairs S (eds): Translational Neurosonology.
Front Neurol Neurosci. Basel, Karger, 2015, vol 36, pp 23–30 (DOI: 10.1159/000366233)

Ultrasound Bio-Effects and Safety Considerations

Gail ter Haar

The Institute of Cancer Research, Sutton, Surrey, UK

Abstract

The responsibility for safe ultrasound applications has been devolved to the user with the introduction of displayed safety indices on the scanner screen. It is therefore essential that the mechanisms of interaction of the ultrasound beam with the tissue being interrogated are properly understood and that the potential biological effects are determined.   © 2015 S. Karger AG, Basel

Introduction

In most people's eyes, diagnostic ultrasound is a safe imaging modality for which there is no need for concern about the risk to the patient under investigation. However, those who are aware of the many therapeutic uses of ultrasound (ranging from the stimulation of bone growth at very low energies to the ablation of tissue for cancer therapy using highly focused high-intensity beams) must be aware that ultrasound energy is capable of producing biological effects in the tissues through which it passes. The area of most concern has been in obstetric ultrasound, and even here, where the rapidly dividing cells of the embryo or fetus are being exposed to ultrasound, the safety record is apparently excellent, with epidemiological studies giving no indication of harm. The only consistent finding has been an increase in the incidence of non-left-handedness in boys exposed in utero [1]. While this epidemiological evidence is reassuring, two things must be borne in mind. First, the children who were the subjects of these studies were exposed to ultrasound in its early days, when the energy outputs from the machines were much lower than they are today. Second, the fact that there is no evidence for harmful effects is not proof that there are no potentially harmful effects occurring; it only means that none has been detected. We know that modern ultrasound scanners are capable of warming tissues in vivo, of applying stress to tissues, and in some circumstances, of damaging structures lying close to gas. In using ultrasound, therefore, it is important to be conversant with the way in which it interacts with tissue and with the potential biological effects that can occur. Armed with this information, it is possible to use ultrasound safely and to best effect, whether diagnostically or for therapy.

The use of ultrasound for neurological applications presents particular challenges. Ultrasound is rapidly attenuated by thin layers of bone, which has two main consequences: local heating at the bone surface and an inability to get ultrasound energy through to tissues lying behind the bone. Techniques such as time reversal (also known as adaptive focusing) are needed to achieve sufficient sound transmission through the skull to provide useful therapy in the brain [2]. Similar techniques can be used to provide ultrasound energy to those abdominal organs lying behind the rib cage [3].

There is a rapidly increasing number of ways in which ultrasonic energy is being used to therapeutic advantage. A number of reviews have reported on these [4–6].

Mechanisms of Interaction

Ultrasound bio-effects result from the interaction between the pressure wave and the tissue through which it passes. Broadly, these interactions can be divided into two types: those that are thermal in origin and those that are non-thermal. Understanding of these interactions is essential if they are to be harnessed (for therapeutic benefit) or avoided (where the concern is for safety).

Thermal Mechanisms

The further an ultrasound wave travels through tissue, the more energy it loses. This loss is known as attenuation and is the result of two processes: scattering and absorption. The physical properties of medical ultrasound mean that it is scattered by the tissue structures that it encounters. This is the basis for ultrasound imaging. Some energy is scattered back at 180°, and some is scattered out of the beam path. Absorption, however, accounts for the majority of attenuation (~60–80%) in soft tissues. Both the incident and the scattered waves contribute to absorption. Tissues have characteristic attenuation and absorption coefficients, with air and bone attenuating ultrasound energy most strongly. Most soft tissues have similar attenuating properties. Attenuation and absorption coefficients are usually quoted in units of dB cm^{-1} MHz^{-1} or nepers cm^{-1} MHz^{-1} (1 neper = 8.68 dB). For soft tissues, attenuation lies between 0.5 and 1.5 dB cm^{-1} MHz^{-1} [7]. Bone is more absorbent than 'soft' tissues, with the brain, for example, having an average absorption coefficient of 0.2 dB cm^{-1} MHz^{-1}

and that of bone being ~10 dB cm^{-1} MHz^{-1} [7]. This means that whereas in soft tissues, the energy is reduced by ~10% in travelling a millimeter, in bone, the reduction is ~85%. At interfaces between different soft tissue types, there is very little reflection of the sound beam, whereas at a bone/soft tissue interface, the majority of the incident beam is reflected, effectively doubling the intensity at the periosteal surface. The temperature rise will thus be greatest at the bone-soft tissue boundary and may give rise to pain from heating of the nerve-rich periosteum. In addition, whereas most soft tissues are well vascularized, thus allowing heat to be carried away from the exposed volume, bone has a relatively poor blood supply. Bone pain may be a limiting factor in physiotherapy treatments and in trans-cranial applications. Pulsed Doppler exposures at maximum output carry the potential for biologically significant temperature rises. In experimental animals, temperature rises in excess of 2°C have been measured close to the skull [8].

In the interests of safety, diagnostic scanners display a safety index related to temperature rises. The thermal index (TI) is intended as an indication of temperature increase, based on which the potential for thermally mediated biological effects can be assessed. The TI is calculated from the source acoustic power divided by the power needed to raise the tissue temperature by 1°C [9]. Three thermal indices are defined: TIS for soft tissues, TIB when bone lies at the beam focus, and TIC for situations in which bone lies close to the surface (the cranial index).

A back-of-the-envelope calculation shows that an intensity of I W cm^{-2} in soft tissue will lead to a temperature that rises at a rate (depending on the product of the absorption coefficient and the intensity) of 0.048°C s^{-1} (2.88°C min^{-1}) at 1 MHz in the absence of cooling factors such as blood flow. At the bone surface, this value may be doubled.

An additional source of heating is provided by the ultrasound transducer itself. The efficiency of transducers, that is, their ability to convert electrical energy into acoustic output, is low, or typically 60–70%, and this can result in heating of the probe front face. This thermal energy is conducted into the tissue with which the transducer is in contact, heating the superficial layers. This may be of particular significance for trans-cranial Doppler examinations.

Acoustic Cavitation

An ultrasonic wave interacts with any small gas bubbles that it encounters in a number of ways. These bubbles may be pre-existing gaseous inclusions, such as might occur in the intestine, they may be intentionally introduced microbubble ultrasound contrast agents (UCAs), or they may be drawn out of solution during the negative-going portion of the pressure wave. A number of different definitions of cavitation exist, but the most usual is the 'formation, growth, and oscillation' of bubbles in an acoustic field [10]. The bubble formation phase is a phenomenon known as 'nucleation'. Once formed, the bubbles grow during successive acoustic cycles until they reach a size that is resonant for the frequency of the ultrasound wave driving them. At 1 MHz, this size is ~1 μm. At resonance, a bubble that has, up until then, been undergoing stable (breathing) oscillations may grow very rapidly and implode, resulting in very high temperatures very locally. This is known as inertial (formerly called collapse) cavitation and is highly destructive to the surrounding tissues. Stably oscillating bubbles (undergoing 'non-inertial' cavitation) create streaming patterns (and hence shear stresses) in the fluid medium surrounding them. This phenomenon is thought to be responsible for the enhancement of drug delivery that is the current subject of extensive research [5]. Acoustic cavitation is a complex phenomenon that has been widely studied and that has been the subject of excellent reviews [11, 12]. Large gas bubbles (e.g. in the bowel) reflect ultrasound strongly, hindering the further transmission of the sound field.

UCAs are designed to scatter ultrasound optimally and thus are also micron sized. Under ultrasonic exposure of sufficient acoustic pressure amplitude, they undergo oscillations and break up, resulting in a hyper-echoic flash on a B-mode image. This is used diagnostically to study bubble kinetics, as it allows visualization of their 'wash in' and 'wash out' of a region of interest.

The use of microbubble contrast agents raises potential safety concerns. While there is no proven evidence of harm resulting from clinical use of these agents, caution is advised when acquiring contrast-enhanced images with mechanical indices (MIs) above 0.4 (see below) since this is the threshold above which in vivo microvascular bio-effects (microvascular rupture and petechial hemorrhage) have been seen in soft tissues [13]. The intra-venous injection of UCAs increases the potential for the hazard associated with gas bodies in tissues exposed to ultrasound. In performing a contrast-enhanced ultrasound scan, the ratio of the risk to the benefit gained must be taken into account. This can be only properly assessed with a good knowledge of available experimental and clinical evidence. While organizations such as the Food and Drug Administration have responsibility for product safety, patient safety remains the responsibility of the clinician, so it is essential that ultrasound users keep themselves informed of safety-related issues. The behavior of these UCAs in ultrasound fields has been comprehensively reviewed. The scientific evidence that biological effects are induced by ultrasound exposures in the presence of UCAs is growing rapidly, although the vast majority of studies have involved exposure of cell cultures in vitro, or model systems that, as discussed below, may have only limited relevance to the in vivo situation. A new and potentially exciting area of research for ultrasound therapy is concerned with the combination of UCAs and low levels of therapeutic ultrasound to transiently open the blood-brain barrier to aid drug delivery [14, 15]. The interaction of ultrasonically driven UCAs and thrombolytic drugs is also being investigated for the treatment of stroke [16, 17].

The display of an MI on modern ultrasound scanners recognizes that bubble activity (in the form of acoustic cavitation) may have important safety implications. This index takes the form

$$MI = p_r/\sqrt{f}$$

where p_r is the local rarefactional pressure in MPa and f is frequency in MHz[9]. When no UCAs are present, the probability of bubble formation in tissue is considered to be low when the MI <1. Common current contrast-enhanced imaging practice is to increase the MI during exposure to destroy the UCAs in the field of view in order to use the imaging of their re-appearance to demonstrate the local vasculature [18].

Conclusions about the safety of the clinical use of UCAs have largely been derived from studies in small rodents. There have been no prospective randomized epidemiological studies to date, although some retrospective analysis of their use in echocardiology has been carried out.

Since the main clinical application of contrast-enhanced ultrasound imaging so far has been in cardiology, it is natural that most published safety studies have concentrated on the heart and skeletal muscle. Here, the most common finding has been of premature ventricular contractions (PVCs). First seen in human volunteers using an MI of 1.5 [19], this finding has since been replicated in rats. The effect was greatest when ultrasound exposures were triggered at end systole in both humans and rodents. A comparison of the induction of PVCs by the three agents – Definity, Albunex, and Optison – in rodent studies found a similar threshold for all agents, but exposures in the presence of Definity resulted in the lowest number of events [20]. A second human study was unable to induce PVCs at MI values ≤1 [21].

Microvessel rupture was first observed in the rat spinotrapezius muscle following ultrasound and UCA exposure using a phased array diagnostic system operating in harmonic imaging mode (2.3 MHz; MI >0.4) [22]. This rupture, as well as the induction of petechiae, has been reported by other investigators in a number of biological models. Clinically insignificant levels of hemolysis (<0.4%) were seen when mouse hearts were exposed through the chest wall (1.15 MHz or 2.23 MHz), and none could be induced in rabbits following exposure to 5 MHz ultrasound (MI of 0.5). The combined effect of ultrasound and UCA exposure on the microvasculature has also been studied in the intestine and kidney, with leakage and petechiae being reported in small animals, but generally has not been replicated in larger animals, such as pigs [13].

Bio-Effects

Many safety studies are initially conducted using individual cell lines maintained in suspension or monolayer cultures. There are a number of advantages to such a system since it allows the study of effects on specific individual cell types and facilitates the detailed characterization of the acoustic field in the exposure chamber containing the cells. However, care must be taken in the interpretation of results obtained with these models since the nutrient media in which the cells are maintained have very low acoustic absorption (typically similar to that of water) and also cavitate more readily than 'solid' tissues. Thus, the relative probability of the mechanism for induction of any bio-effects seen (thermal or cavitational) is reversed compared with that in the in vivo situation. The exposure of cells in suspension culture may result in different effects than those induced in cells growing in monolayers attached to a substrate. In suspension, both cells and microbubbles are free to move, can be in the high-intensity regions of the ultrasonic field only fleetingly, and may not be in close proximity to each other for long. When looking at the effects of UCAs in monolayer cultures, bubbles may be pushed up against the cell layer by the radiation pressure in the beam, thus maximizing the probability of interaction between the cells and the contrast agents. This exposure geometry is in turn very different from that which might be expected during UCA use in vivo. That said, provided that these concerns are properly addressed, useful results can be obtained.

It has been demonstrated that ultrasound exposure in vitro can induce a variety of effects at the cellular level. These range from cell lysis to subtle changes in membrane permeability and ionic transport.

Most in vitro studies involving UCAs have concentrated on effects on red blood cells since these bubbles are primarily used to demonstrate vascularity. The general finding is that the pressure threshold needed to produce hemolysis is significantly reduced in the presence of UCAs [23]. If not destroyed by the ultrasound exposure or passage through the vasculature, UCAs may be taken up by phagocytes in the body. The effect of ultrasound on cells that have phagocytosed such microbubbles has therefore been studied by a number of authors, and it has been found that the threshold for cell membrane disruption is reduced in the presence of contrast agents. Similarly, the threshold for endothelial cell surface changes was reduced when exposures were carried out with UCAs in contact with the cells [23].

Although measurement of the in situ ultrasound field is more difficult in intact tissues, some useful insight into ultrasonically induced bio-effects may be gained from the study of freshly excised tissues. Here, the advantage is that the cells are arranged in the same way as in vivo, with comparable adjacency to other cells and important stromal components. Ex vivo tissues lack an intact blood supply, and care must be taken to use fresh, degassed samples, as gases released by autolysis increase the probability of cavitation events.

Effects resulting from ultrasound exposures in vivo can largely be attributed to a thermal mechanism of action. Heating may result in a number of effects, depending on the temperature rise and the duration of heating. At one extreme, temperatures in excess of 56°C maintained for 1 s or longer will lead to protein denaturation and tissue necrosis [24]. Temperatures in the range of 39–41°C can lead to a stimulation of the local blood supply. Acoustic cavitation is difficult to induce in tissue in the absence of UCAs. The field of histotripsy [25] harnesses cavitation bubble clouds to mechanically destroy tissue regions. Here, short (~5 cycle) pulses with large negative pressure amplitude (~15 MPa) are used. With more conventional ultrasound exposures, cavitation is difficult to induce. Peak negative pressure thresholds for cavitation are quoted in the literature, but these are hugely variable and depend on a wide range of tissue- and transducer-related variables [26]. For most diagnostic applications, cavitation is unlikely to occur.

Mitigating Hazard

The safety indices referred to above are designed to provide guidance for the ultrasound user. The British Medical Ultrasound Society has developed safe-use guidelines that suggest safe times for scan exposures based on minimizing thermal and cavitational damage [27]. These have been endorsed by the European Federation of Societies for Ultrasound in Medicine and Biology. For adult trans-cranial scanning, it is recommended that the trans-cranial thermal index (TIC) be monitored. The guidance recommends that TIC ≥ 3 never be used and that a TIC <1 be used for an indefinite time, provided care is taken and that the ALARA principle is followed. For $1 \leq$ TIC < 1.5, the maximum recommended scan time is 30 min; for $1.5 \leq$ TIC < 2, 15 min; for $2 \leq$ TIC < 2.5, 4 min; and for $2.5 \leq$ TIC < 3, 1 min. When UCAs are used, the guidelines recommend that an MI >0.7 be used with caution. For neonatal trans-cranial scanning, the recommendations are essentially the same, except that the lower level for indefinite scanning is set at 0.7, with $0.7 \leq$ TIC < 1.0 being restricted to 60 min scans. These levels are derived from the World Federation of Societies for Ultrasound in Medicine and Biology statements on thermal effects [28].

References

1 Salvesen KÅ: Ultrasound in pregnancy and non-right handedness: meta-analysis of randomized trials. Ultrasound Obstet Gynecol 2011;38:267–271.

2 Tanter M, Pernot M, Aubry JF, et al: Compensating for bone interfaces and respiratory motion in high-intensity focused ultrasound. Int J Hyperthermia 2007;23:141–151.

3 Aubry J-F, Pernot M, Marquet F, et al: Transcostal high-intensity-focused ultrasound: ex vivo adaptive focusing feasibility study. Phys Med Biol 2008;53: 2937–2951.

4 Monteith S, Sheehan J, Medel R, et al: Potential intracranial applications of magnetic resonance-guided focused ultrasound surgery. J Neurosurg 2013; 118:215–221.

5 Castle J, Butts M, Healey A, et al: Ultrasound-mediated targeted drug delivery: recent success and remaining challenges. Am J Physiol Heart Circ Physiol 2013;304:H350–H357.

6 Malietzis G, Monzon L, Hand J, et al: High-intensity focused ultrasound: advances in technology and experimental trials support enhanced utility of focused ultrasound surgery in oncology. Br J Radiol 2013;86:20130044, DOI: http://dx.doi.org/10.1259/bjr.20130044.

7 Duck FA: Physical Properties of Tissue. A Comprehensive Reference Book. London, UK: Academic Press, 1990.

8 Church CC: Ultrasound-induced heating and its biological consequences; in ter Haar GR (ed): The Safe Use of Ultrasound in Medical Diagnosis. London, BMUS/BIR British Institute of Radiology, 2012.

9 National Council on Radiation Protection and Measurements: Exposure Criteria for Medical Diagnostic Ultrasound: 1. Criteria Based on Thermal Mechanisms. Report no. 113. Bethesda, MD, National Council for Radiation Protection and Measurements, 1992.

10 Leighton T: The Acoustic Bubble. London, Academic Press Limited, 1994.

11 Stride E, Coussios C-C: Cavitation and contrast: the use of bubbles in ultrasound imaging and therapy. Proc Inst Mech Eng H 2010;224:171–191.

12 McLaughlan J, Rivens I, Leighton T, et al: A study of bubble activity generated in ex vivo tissue by high intensity focused ultrasound. Ultrasound Med Biol 2010;36:1327–1344.

13 Miller DL: The safe use of contrast-enhanced diagnostic ultrasound; in ter Haar GR (ed): The Safe Use of Ultrasound in Medical Diagnosis. London, BMUS/BIR British Institute of Radiology, 2012.

14 Kinoshita M, McDannold N, Jolesz F, et al: Targeted delivery of antibodies through the blood-brain barrier by MRI-guided focused ultrasound. Biochem Biophys Res Commun 2006;340:1085–1090.

15 Tung Y-S, Vlachos F, Choi J, et al: In vivo Transcranial cavitation threshold detection during ultrasound-induced blood-brain barrier opening in mice. Phys Med Biol 2010;55:6141–6155.

16 Saqqur M, Tsivgoulis G, Nicoli F, et al: The role of sonolysis and sonothrombolysis in acute ischemic stroke: a systematic review and meta-analysis of randomized controlled trials and case-control studies. J Neuroimaging 2014;24:209–220.

17 Meiars S: Sonothrombolysis.

18 Tang M-X, Mulvana H, Gauthier T, et al: Quantitative contrast-enhanced ultrasound imaging: a review of sources of variability. Interface Focus 2011;1:520–539.

19 van der Wouw P, Brauns AC, Bailey SE, et al: Premature ventricular contractions during triggered imaging with ultrasound contrast. J Am Soc Echocardiogr 2000;13:288–294.

20 Dalecki D, Rota C, Raeman CH, et al: Premature cardiac contractions produced by ultrasound and microbubble contrast agents in mice. Acoust Res Lett Online 2005;6:221–226.

21 Raisinghani A, Wei KS, Crouse L, et al: Myocardial contrast echocardiography (MCE) with triggered ultrasound does not cause premature ventricular complexes: evidence from PB127 MCE studies. J Am Soc Echocardiogr 2003;16:1037–1042.

22 Skyba DM, Price RJ, Linka AZ, et al: Direct in vivo visualization of intravascular destruction of microbubbles by ultrasound and its local effects on tissue. Circulation 1998;98:290–293.

23 Miller D: Overview of experimental studies of biological effects of medical ultrasound caused by gas body activation and inertial cavitation. Prog Biophys Mol Biol 2007;93:314–330.

24 Larson TR, Bostwick DG, Corica A: Temperature-correlated histopathologic changes following microwave thermoablation of obstructive tissue in patients with benign prostatic hyperplasia. Urology 1996;47:463–469.

25 Roberts W: Development and translation of histotripsy: current status and future directions. Curr Opin Urol 2014;24:104–110.

26 Bull V, Civale J, Rivens I, et al: A comparison of acoustic cavitation detection thresholds measured with piezo-electric and fiber-optic hydrophone sensors. Ultrasound Med Biol 2013;39:2406–2421.

27 The British Medical Ultrasound Society: Guidelines for the safe use of diagnostic ultrasound equipment. 2009. http://www.bmus.org/policies-guides/BMUS-Safety-Guidelines-2009-revision-FINAL-Nov-2009.pdf.

28 WFUMB Symposium on Safety of Ultrasound in Medicine. Conclusions and recommendations on thermal and non-thermal mechanisms for biological effects of ultrasound. Kloster-Banz, Germany. 14–19 April, 1996. World Federation for Ultrasound in Medicine and Biology. Ultrasound Med Biol 1998; 24(suppl 1):xv–xvi.

Prof. Gail ter Haar
Division of Radiotherapy and Imaging, Institute of Cancer Research
Royal Marsden Hospital
Sutton, Surrey SM2 5PT (UK)
E-Mail gail.terhaar@icr.ac.uk

Alonso A, Hennerici MG, Meairs S (eds): Translational Neurosonology.
Front Neurol Neurosci. Basel, Karger, 2015, vol 36, pp 31–39 (DOI: 10.1159/000366234)

Intima-Media Thickness of Carotid Arteries

Pierre-Jean Touboul

Stroke Center Bichat Hospital, INSERM U698, Paris, France

Abstract

Carotid intima-media thickness (CIMT) is a validated predictive marker of increased plaque occurrence and the incidence of major cardiovascular events. However, due to technical issues associated with the measurement of CIMT, a well-trained and certified sonographer is needed to overcome causes of variability due to the patient, device, sonographer, and quantification tool. The recently updated Mannheim consensus defined and described how to differentiate CIMT from plaques. These definitions allow for the better analysis and quantification of early atherosclerosis. Indications for CIMT measurements largely include the detection of coronary heart disease risk among intermediate-risk patients. CIMT is frequently used in clinical trials, and recent technical recommendations have been provided to improve the quality of the procedures. The final choice of a CIMT protocol depends on the purpose of the measurement, the research question at hand, the cost effectiveness, the quality of the data and the added value provided by the additional information.

Introduction

Symptomatic cardiovascular disease generally occurs when atherosclerosis blocks blood flow, causing ischemia, or when a thrombus forms on a plaque as a result of rupture or of erosion. When a clinical event occurs, the atherosclerotic disease is difficult to reverse [1]. Therefore, the prevention of the development of atherosclerosis or of its progression has become an important goal in medicine to reduce cardiovascular death and morbidity. In 1986, Pignoli published the first paper on the relation between common carotid intima-media histology and a double-line pattern identified as the intima-media complex detected at the same site with ultrasound [1]. Since that time, the ultrasonography of carotid arteries has become a frequently used method to detect early signs of atherosclerosis, i.e., the increased thickness of the arterial wall or plaque occurrence. It is a safe, non-expensive, feasible and accurate method. An increased carotid intima-media thickness (CIMT) does not immediately lead to cardio-

Table 1. Human and device factors of variability of IMT measurement

Patient	Device	Sonographer	Measurement
Age	Frequency	Education	Manual
Tissue echogenicity	Grey scale	Far wall	Semi-automatic
Neck anatomy	Depth settings	CCA/C.Bif/OICA	Real-time
Risk factors	Gain settings	Left/right	Software
Race	Frame rate	Plaque/no plaque	Mean/max.
Gender	RF/video	Number of angles	Points or segment (10 mm)
Country			Cardiac cycle

vascular events but reflects the degree of atherosclerosis elsewhere in the arterial system [2]. When CIMT is measured at several time points within an individual, the rate of change in CIMT can also be calculated. Both measures reflect cardiovascular disease risk and have been used as a surrogate marker in clinical trials. The first cohort studies reported relations between cardiovascular risk factors and CIMT [3–6], after which the predictive value of CIMT on cardiovascular events was established [7]. Additionally, the rate of change in CIMT has been under investigation in trials [8–10] and cohort studies [11, 12].

Technical Issues in Carotid Intima-Media Thickness Ultrasound Evaluation

CIMT measurements are not the same; each separate CIMT value has its own absolute value, reproducibility, obtainable completeness, rate of change over time and relation with cardiovascular events [13–15]. Variability in the absolute CIMT value can be attributed to various factors, including the characteristics of the patient, the device used, the sonographer and the measurement approach (table 1).

Ultrasound Examination of the Patient

The CIMT measurement is obtained when the patient is in the supine position, with a slight rotation of the neck to the contralateral side with the minimal tension of the cervical muscles. Images are best obtained with linear/array transducers with high-resolution probes at frequencies ≥7 MHz. Measurements are best acquired at the end of the diastole because the systolic expansion of the lumen causes the CIMT to become thinner. Image resolution depends on the settings (gain and depth), frame rate and device. CIMT acquisition needs a depth setting of between 35 and 45 mm, which is usually 40 mm. Gain settings should be adjusted to avoid the overexposure or underexposure of the near and far walls. Time gain control may be important to adjust to decrease arterial lumen artefacts. Wall thickness depends on the anatomical location due to shear stress, which varies according to flow direction [14, 16]. At the bifurcation, the angle, the diameter of the bulb and the curvature of the origin of the internal carotid artery may induce remodelling, which increases the inter-individual variability of IMT at these sites. Apart from the device aspects, the absolute CIMT value depends heavily on patient characteristics as recently reviewed by Peters and coworkers [17].

Sonographer

Image acquisition is the main factor causing the variability of the ultrasound examination, which depends on the education and experience of the sonographer. Recommendations on CIMT acquisition and measurement have been published and updated for carotid image acquisition [14, 15]. However, there is no standard for the training and certification of sonographers and readers. A programme for training has been published; however, it has not been implemented in a systematic manner [17, 18]. At the least, the sonographers and readers should be trained to perform measurements and interpret findings. It has also been recommended to obtain estimates of the variabilities of the sonographers before and repeatedly during the studies. Groups that work with CIMT measurements should document their accuracy and reproducibility to assure that they are similar to those reported in the literature [16]. Some devices are equipped with an online quality index, which provides a measure of success based on the quality of image acquisition when used in real time [19].

Acquisition of Ultrasound Images for Carotid Intima-Media Thickness Measurements

Ultrasound protocols to measure CIMT may vary in the selections of the carotid segments, angles, and walls of the carotid artery measured. Measurements can be done on the near wall and/or the far wall along the common carotid artery, the carotid bifurcation and/or the internal carotid artery at one or more angles of insonation (anterior, lateral and posterior). Some protocols measure only at the far wall of the common carotid segment using one image, whereas other protocols measure at the common carotid artery, the internal carotid artery and the bifurcation. The near wall is more difficult to delimitate, particularly at the posterior and anterior regions. In vitro experiments have shown that the far-wall CIMT best reflects the true thickness of the arterial wall, based on the properties of the ultrasound waves [20]. The near wall represents at best an approximation of the true wall thickness. Furthermore, it is generally thought that near-wall CIMT measurements are more difficult to obtain. Therefore, the two consensuses recommend far-wall measurements, which can be acquired successfully in almost all patients [14, 15]. However, near-wall measurements can be readily and easily measured in many situations. Additionally, the near wall or the combination of the near- and far-wall measurements can be measured very reproducibly. In trials, the combination of near- and far-wall measurements have been shown to be superior to far-wall measurements alone [14, 21]. This is partially because random error is reduced when the number of measurements is increased and averaged [22]. Thus, when possible, near-wall measurements combined with far-wall data may provide valuable information. The choice made to analyse both walls should, of course, also depend on the time invested for acquisition in relation to the scientific benefit.

Because atherosclerosis is an asymmetric disease, CIMT and its progression differs among the carotid segments [14, 23–25]. The carotid bifurcation and internal carotid artery, which is next to the common carotid artery, may carry additional information on atherosclerotic disease [14–16, 26]. In addition, the heterogeneity of the relationships between cardiovascular risk factors and CIMT measurements at different carotid segments and walls is another argument in favour of a more extensive ultrasound protocol [27]. Therefore, depending on the aim of the patient examination, the ultrasound protocol can be restricted to the far wall of the common carotid artery or extended to the whole carotid tree.

In 3,364 individuals in whom the carotid artery was systematically examined using the same extensive ultrasound protocol, an asymmetric circumferential pattern of atherosclerosis was observed in both men and women, the young and old, among different race groups, and across the four participating studies [16]. The asymmetrical helix-like distribution of atherosclerosis in the carotid arteries expands the evidence by showing that the atherosclerotic configuration is similar across populations with different vascular risks and across genders, ages, and races [16]. These findings show that, particularly for the carotid bifurcation and bulb, the angle of interrogation of the ultrasound beam is an important determinant of the absolute value of the maximum CIMT. This finding implies that carotid ultrasound studies investigating maximum CIMT should include measurements from multiple carotid angles when the bifurcation bulb and the origin of the carotid artery are evaluated.

CIMT and carotid plaques are biologically and genetically distinct phenotypes of atherosclerosis. The definition of plaque may seem clear-cut, yet among observers, differences exist in what is consider to be a plaque, even after training. An accepted definition of an atherosclerotic plaque is a focal thickening of the intima-media complex encroaching into the arterial lumen by at least 0.5 mm or involving 50% of the surrounding IMT, or a focal thickening from the intima-lumen interface to the media-adventitia interface of over 1.5 mm [14]. CIMT and plaques may reflect different aspects of the atherosclerotic process and are differentially related to risk factors and cardiovascular disease. Studies that have separated increased CIMT and plaques have shown a greater risk for myocardial infarction with plaques [28]. The main advantage of measuring CIMT is that it can even be assessed in children and young adults, whereas plaques are mainly present at older ages.

Carotid Intima-Media Thickness Measurement

The most common and basic CIMT measurements are the mean common CIMT and the mean maximum common CIMT. The mean common CIMT is the mean value of the elementary CIMT measurements that are performed over a 10-mm part of the far wall or over both the far and near wall of the common carotid artery. This can represent the mean of 100–150 values. The mean maximum CIMT is calculated as the mean of the single maximum CIMT measurements that are measured from different segments of the carotid artery and is most often used for carotid atherosclerosis evaluations in clinical trials. When plaques are present in a segment, the maximal value is by definition at the maximum height of the plaque.

In most studies, CIMT is read from images using a reading programme, by which the reader can manually draw lines to quantify the IMT or use a semi-automated edge detection programme for assistance with drawing these lines. The associations of CIMT with risk factors and risks for future events have been reported to be stronger for manual than for automated readings in only one study [29]. However, automated reading is more strongly associated with future events in participants with a thinner common CIMT. These findings suggest that a manual approach might be preferred in populations with high prevalences of atherosclerotic burden, whereas an automated approach might be favoured in settings with more easily detectable CIMTs. In 43 healthy women, studies of the reproducibility of automated and manual CIMT measurements of the common carotid artery, carotid bifurcation, and internal carotid artery resulted in reliable CIMT readings across all carotid segments, although the measurement error was lower and the repeatability of the measurements was higher for the automated technique [30]. In the METEOR study, both manual and semi-automated edge detection of the lumen and wall interfaces for the measurement of maximal far-wall common CIMT resulted in high reproducibility, and they further showed largely similar relations to cardiovascular risk factors, rates of change, and treatment effects [31]. It seems that the choice between automated and manual reading software for CIMT studies should be based on logistical and cost considerations rather than differences in data quality.

Normal Carotid Intima-Media Thickness Values

What values of CIMT are 'normal' depends on the population and what is meant by CIMT. Generally, CIMT is perceived as common carotid IMT, yet this needs to be clearly stated. Common CIMT values are reported to be higher in men than in women [32]. Additionally, African-American people have higher values than Caucasians. In general, normal values for common CIMT are thought to be around 0.5 mm in young adults and 1.2 mm in the elderly [15]. Additionally, these values depend on age, gender, risk factor prevalence, echogenicity, the segment, the measurement algorithm, and the ultrasound device. In its 2008 consensus statement, the American Society of Echocardiography suggested that CIMT values at or above the 75th percentile of a reference population indicate increased cardiovascular risk [15]. Currently, several initiatives have been launched to combine existing cohorts worldwide to come up with some estimates of normal values, in which adjustments for equipment and reader algorithms can be taken into account.

Carotid Intima-Media Thickness and Cardiovascular Risk Prediction

Currently, cardiovascular risk prediction in asymptomatic individuals is based on the level of cardiovascular risk factors incorporated into scoring equations [33]. Several scores are available, and the Framingham risk score is among the most widely used [33, 34]. CIMT has been proposed to be added as a cardiovascular risk factor to improve individual risk assessment [8, 35]. So far, individual studies have reported on the added value of CIMT measurements in cardiovascular risk prediction, but the evidence is not consistent across studies [26, 36–39]. This may be attributed to differences in CIMT measurement, in the distribution of age and gender, in the number of events, in the cut-off values for the risk categories and in the endpoint definition [36–39]. Therefore, the guidelines differ in their recommendations to use CIMT measurements in primary prevention and also for whom these measurements should be considered, ranging from measurements in all individuals [40] to measurements in only those at intermediate risk [41]. The recently published Appropriate Use Criteria states that indications for CIMT measurements largely include the detection of coronary heart disease risk among intermediate-risk patients, those with metabolic syndrome and older patients [35]. On-going studies may provide guidance on this topic.

Carotid Intima-Media Thickness in Clinical Trials

CIMT is often used in clinical trials as a surrogate endpoint for cardiovascular events, with the idea that the regression or the slowed progression of CIMT, as induced by cardiovascular drugs, reflects a reduction in these events. The continuous nature of CIMT makes it logical to assume that this linear relationship indeed exists. However, evidence that changes in CIMT directly reflect changes in cardiovascular event risks is inconsistent. One recent meta-analysis on this topic using aggregate data pooled from the literature has shown that changes in CIMT do not reflect a reduction in these events [42]. A second recent meta-analysis using a similar approach and using the same data has shown that the slowed progression of CIMT over time is associated with a lower likelihood of nonfatal myocardial infarction in selected trials but that findings have been inconsistent at times, suggesting caution in using CIMT as a surrogate end point [43]. However, both studies should be interpreted with caution because they both may suffer from considerable flaws as reviewed in detail elsewhere [44]. Besides ecological fallacy, flaws may include heterogeneity in treatment efficacy, patient populations and the methodology of measuring CIMT in addition to a lack of power [44]. An individual participant data analysis is needed to overcome the flaws of these earlier meta-analyses using aggregated data.

Current Technical Recommendations for Carotid Intima-Media Thickness Measurement and Recommended Protocols

In spite of the tremendous increase in the use of CIMT in cardiovascular research, there are no international guidelines on how this technique should be applied as a research tool. Two consensus reports have touched upon this topic; the first was the Mannheim consensus, which was organised in 2004 and updated in 2006 and 2011 [14]. The second was published in 2008 by the American Society of Echocardiography [15]. Both recommend CIMT to be measured preferably at the far wall. The key is of course that the final choice for a certain protocol should be entirely driven by the research question to be answered and not primarily by a consensus protocol. Recent protocols include information regarding the common, bulb and internal carotid segments and a separate measurement of focal plaque. These protocols are feasible and reproducible when strict quality control is ensured. The choice of an ultrasound protocol should depend on the research question, with a well-considered balance between time and cost on the one hand, and data quality and the value of the additional information obtained using extensive protocols on the other.

Summary

CIMT is a validated marker of cardiovascular risk factors, and it predicts the occurrence of cardiovascular events in large populations. The technical issues underlying the current best practice must be known and applied to provide reliable data in clinical practice and trials.

When CIMT measurements are used for cardiovascular research purposes or in clinical practice, strict attention needs to be paid to quality control in acquisition, measurement and interpretation. The final choice of a CIMT protocol should depend on the purpose of the measurement, the research question at hand and the balance between cost, data quality and the value of additional information.

References

1 Pignoli P, Tremoli E, Poli A, et al: Intimal plus medial thickness of the arterial wall: a direct measurement with ultrasound imaging. Circulation 1986;6: 1399–1406.

2 Bots ML, Baldassarre D, Simon A, et al: Carotid intima-media thickness and coronary atherosclerosis: weak or strong relations? Eur Heart J 2007;28:398–406.

3 O'Leary DH, Polak JF, Kronmal RA, et al: Carotid-artery intima and media thickness as a risk factor for myocardial infarction and stroke in older adults. Cardiovascular Health Study Collaborative Research Group. N Engl J Med 1999;340:14–22.

4 Chambless LE, Heiss G, Shahar E, et al: Prediction of ischemic stroke risk in the atherosclerosis risk in Communities Study. Am J Epidemiol 2004;160:259–269.

5 Chambless LE, Folsom AR, Sharrett AR, et al: Coronary heart disease risk prediction in the atherosclerosis risk in communities (ARIC) study. J Clin Epidemiol 2003;56:880–890.

6 Bots ML, Hoes AW, Koudstaal PJ, et al: Common carotid intima-media thickness and risk of stroke and myocardial infarction: the Rotterdam Study. Circulation 1997;96:1432–1437.

7 Lorenz MW, Markus HS, Bots ML, et al: Prediction of clinical cardiovascular events with carotid intima-media thickness: a systematic review and meta-analysis. Circulation 2007;115:459–467.

8 Espeland M, O'Leary DH, Terry J, et al: Carotid intimal-media thickness as a surrogate for cardiovascular disease events in trials of HMG-CoA reductase inhibitors. Curr Control Trials Cardiovasc Med 2005;6:3.

9 Yokoyama H, Katakami N, Yamasaki Y: Recent advances of intervention to inhibit progression of carotid intima-Media thickness in patients with Type 2 diabetes mellitus. Stroke 2006;37:2420–2427.

10 Wang JG, Staessen JA, Li Y, et al: Carotid intima-media thickness and antihypertensive treatment: a meta-analysis of randomized controlled trials. Stroke 2006;37:1933–1940.

11 Chambless LE, Folsom AR, Davis V, et al: Risk factors for progression of common carotid atherosclerosis: the Atherosclerosis Risk in Communities Study, 1987–1998. Am J Epidemiol 2002;155:38–47.

12 van der Meer IM, Iglesias del Sol A, Hak AE, et al: Risk factors for progression of atherosclerosis measured at multiple sites in the arterial tree: the Rotterdam Study. Stroke 2003;34:2374–2379.

13 Dogan S, Duivenvoorden R, Grobbee DE, et al: Ultrasound protocols to measure carotid intima-media thickness in trials; comparison of reproducibility, rate of progression, and effect of intervention in subjects with familial hypercholesterolemia and subjects with mixed dyslipidemia. Ann Med 2010;6:447–464.

14 Touboul PJ, Hennerici MG, Meairs S, et al: Mannheim carotid intima-media thickness and plaque consensus (2004–2006–2011). An update on behalf of the advisory board of the 3rd, 4th and 5th watching the risk symposia, at the 13th, 15th and 20th European Stroke Conferences, Mannheim, Germany, 2004, Brussels, Belgium, 2006, and Hamburg, Germany, 2011. Cerebrovasc Dis 2012;34:290–296.

15 Stein JH, Korcarz CE, Hurst RT, et al: Use of carotid ultrasound to identify subclinical vascular disease and evaluate cardiovascular disease risk: a consensus statement from the American Society of Echocardiography Carotid Intima-Media Thickness Task Force. Endorsed by the Society for Vascular Medicine. J Am Soc Echocardiogr 2008;21:93–111.

16 Tajik P, Meijer R, Duivenvoorden RL, et al: Asymmetrical distribution of atherosclerosis in the carotid artery: identical patterns across age, race, and gender. Eur J Prev Cardiol 2012;19:687–697.

17 Peters SA, Grobbee DE, Bots ML: Carotid intima-media thickness: a suitable alternative for cardiovascular risk as outcome? Eur J Cardiovasc Prev Rehabil 2011;18:167–174.

18 Berglund G, Riley W, Barnes R, et al: Quality control in ultrasound studies on atherosclerosis. J Intern Med 1994;5:581–586.

19 Touboul P-J, Vicaut E, Labreuche J, et al: Design, baseline characteristics and carotid intima-media thickness reproducibility in the PARC study. Cerebrovasc Dis 2005;19:57–63.

20 Wong M, Edelstein J, Wollman J, et al: Ultrasonic-pathological comparison of the human arterial wall. Verification of intima-media thickness. Arterioscler Thromb 1993;13:482–486.

21 Dogan S, Plantinga Y, Crouse III J Jr, et al: Algorithms to measure carotid intima-media thickness in trials: a comparison of reproducibility, rate of progression and treatment effect. J Hypertens 2011;11: 2181–2193.

22 Espeland M, Craven T, Riley W, et al: Reliability of longitudinal ultrasonographic measurements of carotid intimal-medial thicknesses. Asymptomatic Carotid Artery Progression Study Research Group. Stroke 1996;3:480–485.

23 Crouse III JR, Byington RP, Bond MG, et al: Pravastatin, lipids, and atherosclerosis in the carotid arteries (PLAC-II). Am J Cardiol 1995;75:455–459.

24 Espeland MA, Evans GW, Wagenknecht LE, et al: Site-specific progression of carotid artery intimal-medial thickness. Atherosclerosis 2003;171:137–143.

25 Crouse JR, Raichlen JS, Riley WA, et al: Effect of rosuvastatin on progression of carotid intima-media thickness in low-risk individuals with subclinical atherosclerosis: the METEOR Trial. JAMA 2007; 297:1344–1353.

26 Polak JF, Pencina MJ, Pencina KM, et al: Carotid-wall intima-media thickness and cardiovascular events. N Engl J Med 2011;365:213–221.

27 Espeland MA, Tang R, Terry JG, et al: Associations of risk factors with segment-specific intimal-medial thickness of the extracranial carotid artery. Stroke 1999;30:1047–1055.

28 Nguyen-Thanh HT, Benzaquen BS: Screening for subclinical coronary artery disease measuring carotid intima media thickness. Am J Cardiol 2009;104: 1383–1388.

29 Dogan S, Plantinga Y, Dijk JM, et al: Manual B-mode versus automated radio-frequency carotid intima-media thickness measurements. J Am Soc Echocardiogr 2009;22:1137–1144.

30 Freire C, Ribeiro A, Barbosa F, et al: Comparison between automated and manual measurements of carotid intima-media thickness in clinical practice. Vasc Health Risk Manag 2009;5:811–817.

31 Peters SAE, Den Ruijter HM, Palmer MK, et al: Manual or semi-automated edge detection of the maximal far wall common carotid intima-media thickness: a direct comparison. J Intern Med 2012;271: 247–256.

32 Touboul PJ, Labreuche J, Vicaut E, et al: Country-based reference values and impact of cardiovascular risk factors on carotid intima-media thickness in a French population: the 'Paroi Artérielle et Risque Cardio-Vasculaire' (PARC) study. Cerebrovasc Dis 2009;27:361–367.

33 Berger JS, Jordan C, Lloyd-Jones D, et al: Screening for cardiovascular risk in asymptomatic patients. J Am Coll Cardiol 2010;55:1169–1177.

34 D'Agostino RB Sr, Vasan RS, Pencina MJ, et al: General cardiovascular risk profile for use in primary care: the Framingham heart study. Circulation 2008; 117:743–753.

35 The Society of Atherosclerosis Imaging and Prevention: Appropriate use criteria for carotid intima media thickness testing. Atherosclerosis 2011;214:43–46.

36 Elias-Smale SE, Kavousi M, Verwoert GC, et al: Common carotid intima-media thickness in cardiovascular risk stratification of older people: the Rotterdam Study. Eur J Prev Cardiol 2012;19:698–705.

37 Lorenz MW, Schaefer C, Steinmetz H, et al: Is carotid intima media thickness useful for individual prediction of cardiovascular risk? Ten-year results from the Carotid Atherosclerosis Progression Study (CAPS). Eur Heart J 2010;31:2041–2048.

38 Nambi V, Chambless L, Folsom AR, et al: Carotid intima-media thickness and presence or absence of plaque improves prediction of coronary heart disease risk: the ARIC (Atherosclerosis Risk in Communities) study. J Am Coll Cardiol 2010;55:1600–1607.

39 Xie W, Wu Y, Wang W, et al: A longitudinal study of carotid plaque and risk of ischemic cardiovascular disease in the Chinese population. J Am Soc Echocardiogr 2011;7:729–737.

40 Naghavi M, Falk E, Hecht HS, et al: From vulnerable plaque to vulnerable patient – part III: Executive summary of the screening for heart attack prevention and education (SHAPE) task force report. Am J Cardiol 2006;98:2H–15H.

41 Greenland P, Alpert JS, Beller GA, et al: 2010 ACCF/AHA Guideline for Assessment of Cardiovascular Risk in Asymptomatic Adults: Executive Summary. Circulation 2010;122:2748–2764.

42 Costanzo P, Perrone-Filardi P, Vassallo E, et al: Does carotid intima-media thickness regression predict reduction of cardiovascular events? A meta-analysis of 41 randomized trials. J Am Coll Cardiol 2010;56: 2006–2020.

43 Goldberger ZD, Valle JA, Dandekar VK, et al: Are changes in carotid intima-media thickness related to risk of nonfatal myocardial infarction? A critical review and meta-regression analysis. Am Heart J 2010; 160:701–714.

44 Taylor AJ, Bots ML, Kastelein JJP: Vascular disease: meta-regression of CIMT trials-data in, garbage out. Nat Rev Cardiol 2011;8:128–130.

Prof. Pierre-Jean Touboul
Stroke Center Bichat Hospital, INSERM U698
46, rue Henri-Huchard
FR–75018 Paris (France)
E-Mail pjtw@noos.fr

Alonso A, Hennerici MG, Meairs S (eds): Translational Neurosonology.
Front Neurol Neurosci. Basel, Karger, 2015, vol 36, pp 40–56 (DOI: 10.1159/000366236)

Functional TCD: Regulation of Cerebral Hemodynamics – Cerebral Autoregulation, Vasomotor Reactivity, and Neurovascular Coupling

Marc E. Wolf

Department of Neurology, Universitätsmedizin Mannheim, University of Heidelberg, Mannheim, Germany

Abstract

Three main mechanisms influence cerebral hemodynamics, with the aim of adapting the cerebral blood flow to the metabolic demand of the brain. Cerebral autoregulation ensures stable perfusion of the brain, independent of the systemic blood pressure. Vasomotor reactivity reflects the hemodynamic responses to modifications of the arterial pCO_2/pH of the brain tissue. Neurovascular coupling adapts the perfusion to increased metabolic demand as a consequence of enhanced brain activity to permit reasonable functioning of cells. Different methods using transcranial Doppler sonography have been developed to characterize these mechanisms in healthy subjects and under pathologic conditions. The most established applications in clinical settings are described, and the results of specific research studies are briefly reported. © 2015 S. Karger AG, Basel

Introduction

Three main mechanisms influence cerebral hemodynamics, with the aim of adapting the cerebral blood flow (CBF) to the metabolic demand of the brain. The goal of all of these mechanisms is to provide the necessary amount of oxygen to the brain tissue in situations of systemically decreased blood flow or increased demand during enhanced brain activity. This chapter will focus on hemodynamic mechanisms, as illustrated in figure 1:

(1) Cerebral autoregulation ensures stable perfusion of the brain, independent of the systemic blood pressure (within a certain range).

(2) Vasomotor reactivity adapts hemodynamics to the arterial pCO_2/pH of the tissue, which reflects its need for oxygen.

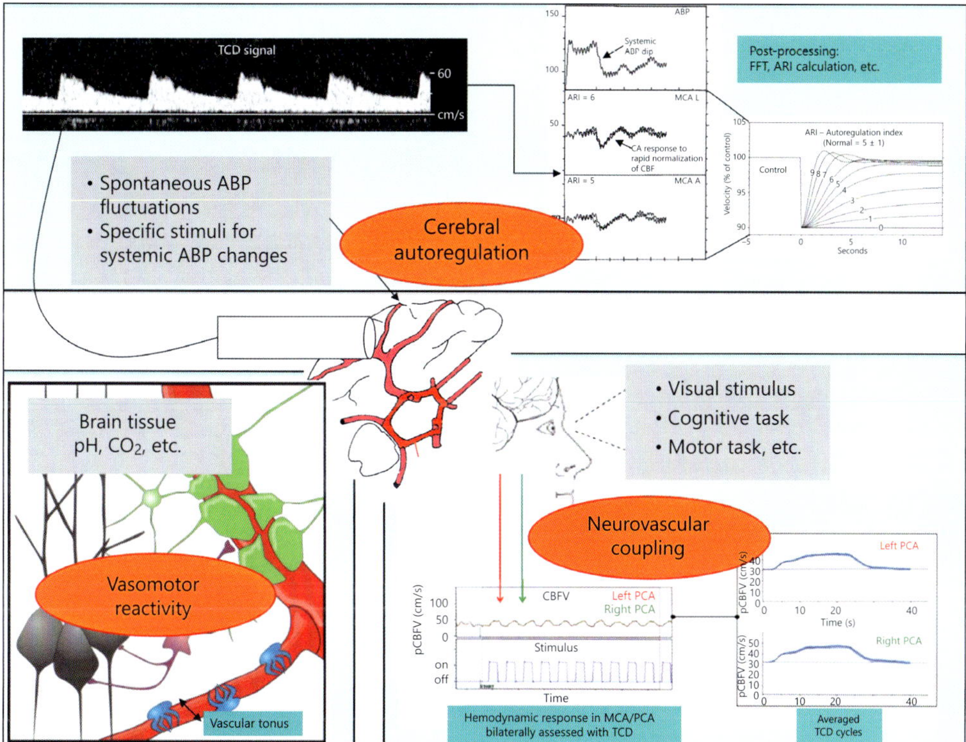

Fig. 1. Illustration of hemodynamic mechanisms influencing cerebral blood flow: cerebral autoregulation, vasomotor reactivity, and neurovascular coupling.

(3) Neurovascular coupling (NVC) adapts the perfusion to increased metabolic demand as a consequence of enhanced brain activity.

The changes in CBF underlying these mechanisms can be recorded and analyzed with functional transcranial Doppler sonography (fTCD), which not only assesses the blood flow velocities of the cerebral vessels but also considers the changes in and reaction of the vasculature induced by external or internal stimuli under normal or pathologic conditions, with a high temporal resolution.

As physiologic background, the diameter of the intracranial vessels is assumed to be stable under different conditions. Therefore, an increase in the CBF velocity (CBFV) reflects an elevation of CBF, the parameter of interest.

First, some general comments about fTCD: Major strengths are its high temporal resolution, the non-invasiveness of the technique, the possibility of using it even at beside (e.g. in intensive care units (ICUs) or actually during surgery), and its relatively easy handling. This entails the possibility of performing follow-up investigations. For the patient, the test procedure is not very stressful compared with competing techniques such as fMRI. In general, the costs are affordable. However, one should be aware of some weaknesses. The technique has a low spatial resolution, and no direct anatomical image is procured. The measurements reflect relative differences (inter-hemispheric comparisons or maximum vs. minimum) rather than absolute values, and the recording and interpretation are somehow operator dependent. Some patients are not assessable due to an insufficient bone window, and some might have pathologies (e.g. intracranial vascular stenosis or systemic disorders such as anemia or cardiac pathologies) affecting the results of the TCD.

The aim of this book is to focus on the translational aspects of ultrasound. Therefore, an effort was made to include the results of animal studies, when possible. However, since fTCD may be applied in humans without affecting their health, experimental studies are scarce, and studies in humans are more appropriate to characterize the respective mechanisms.

Given the large number of different methods, evaluation systems, and clinical studies in this field, the discussion of some aspects needed to be shortened or omitted. This is not always mentioned explicitly. However, an effort was made to provide additional references to give the reader the opportunity to further deepen his knowledge of issues in which he is specifically interested.

Cerebral Autoregulation

Definition

Cerebral autoregulation (CA) accounts for the stabilization of cerebral perfusion in the presence of systemic hypo- or hypertension. For mean systemic arterial blood pressures (ABPs) between 50–60 and 150–170 mm Hg (and the respective cerebral perfusion pressures, or CPPs), the CBF is kept constant. Above and below these limits, the mechanism does not evolve reasonably, entailing potentially harmful hypo- or hyperperfusion of the brain tissue.

The regulation is based on cerebrovascular resistance (CVR) and is mainly adjusted in the small arterioles and precapillary sphincters. Three mechanisms play a role: metabolic regulation, mediated by the release of vasoactive substances, when oxygen is needed; myogenic regulation, mediated by adapting the vascular tone to the transmural blood pressure (BP); and neurogenic regulation, mediated by sympathetic innervation of the vascular smooth cells.

One can distinguish between two types of CA. Static CA adapts the CBF to slow/gradual changes in ABP within minutes or hours. This dates back to the pre-fTCD era since available methods needed to average several minutes of recording. With the high temporal resolution of fTCD, dynamic cerebral autoregulation (dCA), responding to immediate ABP changes within seconds, can be analyzed by considering the beat-to-beat dynamics.

CA and CBF show some variations related to daytime, exercise, forced respiration (with changes in the arterial pCO_2), body position, and functional activation. Food intake, caffeine intake, and hormonal changes like the menstrual cycle also play a role. These fluctuations have to be kept in mind for standardization when performing CA tests either in a cohort (to evaluate each patient under the same conditions) or in intra-individual longitudinal studies. One should also consider the influence of anesthetics [1].

Animal Studies

Animal studies have been published since the 1960s. Most of them have used different techniques, such as electromagnetic flowmetry (see review by Panerai) [2]. Precursor studies of the carotid compression test have been performed in monkeys. CA studies with concomitant intracerebral pressure (ICP) measurements have been performed in piglet brains. Impaired CA in hypertensive rats has been associated with larger ischemic lesions in experimental stroke models.

With the development of fTCD, direct non-invasive investigation of human subjects was possible. Autoregulation seems to be more important in humans, who are subjected to severe orthostatic stresses more than quadrupeds are. Therefore, the mechanisms might differ.

Methods in Humans

Stimulation Techniques

Evaluation of static CA has mostly been performed using pharmacological interventions to achieve gradual changes in ABP.

Several techniques using a stimulus-response method have been established to assess and quantify dCA. The dynamics of the CBFV after a rapid ABP drop (and the time until the CBFV reaches steady state again) are considered. Simple or oscillatory stimuli are used. For further details, see the review by Panerai [2].

The leg-cuff method (Aaslid et al. [3]) involves the perfusion of both proximal lower extremities being blocked for 2–3 min with a BP cuff (> the systemic pressure), followed by rapid deflation. This entails a rapid step-wise systemic decrease in the ABP (by about 20 mm Hg) and should activate an increase in the CBFV of 20%/s under normal conditions.

Contraindications are a vascular disease or fracture of the leg and, in general, an unstable ICP [4]. The stimulus might not represent the typical physiologic situation in daily life (e.g. changes in posture or pharmacological stimuli due to medication). However, the test is performed in a supine position, and therefore, bedfast patients can be investigated.

The carotid artery compression test/transient hyperemic response [5] involves the common carotid artery being compressed within the neck as low as possible. With a

CBFV decrease of 30–50%, compression is considered as sufficient, and after 3 s, the compression is released in the diastole. This manipulation induces a 'transient hyperemic response' (THR) with a compensatory vasodilatation of the arterioles. The response can be quantified according to the 'transient hyperemic response ratio' (THRR):

$$\text{THRR} = \frac{v_{hyperemic}}{v_{basic}}$$

($v_{hyperemic}$ = the systolic CBFV 2 cycles after compression release; v_{basic} = the systolic CBFV 5 cycles before compression).

Normal values vary between 1.105 and 1.29. There is a risk of generating emboli, and the test is very uncomfortable for patients, limiting its repeatability.

The Valsalva maneuver (expiration against a 30 mm Hg pressure for 15 s) can induce ABP changes and accordingly CA responses [6]. However, the increase in the intrathoracic pressure also leads to an elevation of the ICP, which additionally reduces the CPP. Another disturbing factor that might influence CA is the increase in end-tidal CO_2. Regular slow respiration is another useful method, but again, it entails the risk of increasing tidal volumes and inducing hypocapnia during the test.

The 'sit-to-stand technique' reflects a relatively physiologic condition of an ABP decrease, consisting of 2 cycles of sitting for 5 min (with legs elevated at 90°) and 1 min of standing, followed by 5 min of sitting and standing again [7]. The method has recently been validated in comparison with the leg-cuff test, showing similar responses [8]. Other methods to induce ABP oscillations are periodic squatting, a passive head-up tilt test, isometric handgrip exercises (the patient needs to cooperate), and a cold pressure test. A more sophisticated technique is the application of a sinusoidal lower-body negative pressure, which entails periodic variations of the ABP. The negative pressure leads to distribution of the blood in the lower extremities and an ABP drop [9]. The procedure is uncomfortable and not possible in obese patients. Some authors have criticized lower-body negative pressure as potentially inducing CA impairment itself.

In contrast to externally induced CA responses, spontaneous dCA reflects adaptation to internally triggered CBF fluctuations. Recording of such spontaneous oscillations of ABP and CBF became popular in the 1990s. Post-processing analysis by complex algorithms and longer recording times are required.

One can distinguish between two spectrums of oscillations: low-frequency oscillations (LFOs), also called Mayer waves (M-waves) and very-low-frequency oscillations (VLFOs), also known as B-waves. LFOs probably reflect changes in sympathetic tone and would be driven by spontaneous mean ABP changes, whereas VLFOs seem to reflect spontaneous oscillations of the ICP and would be triggered by other mechanisms.

Data Quantification

Several approaches have been used to characterize CA. A comprehensive overview of exemplary indices is given in a review by van Beek et al. [10]. Based on the assumption of a linear relationship, several scores have been developed, including CVR:

$$CVR = \frac{mean\ BP}{mean\ CBF}\ [mm\ Hg/ml/min].$$

In TCD studies, the CVR index (CVRi) can be used:

$$CVRi = \frac{mean\ BP}{mean\ CBFV}\ [mm\ Hg/cm/s].$$

Goslings' pulsatility index (PI) is a common tool used to characterize the vasomotor resistance and correlates with the CVR under steady-state conditions. However, the PI seems less useful for CA characterization since it does not always react in the same way as the CVR when conditions change [10].

$$PI = \frac{CBFVsys - CBFVdias}{mean\ CBFV}.$$

Another way to characterize CA is linear extrapolation of the value of ABP at which the CBF would approach zero. This is called the critical closing pressure (in mm Hg).

More sophisticated characterization of dCA is a time or frequency domain analysis. The autoregulation index (ARI) (Tiecks et al. [11]) evaluates the time domain. As technical background, the CBFV is assumed to passively follow the ABP decrease. A computer-based system fits a potential curve to this condition. If the measured curve fits with this model, the ARI is zero, reflecting no autoregulation response. Nine other curves are generated, with increasingly better adaptation to the ABP decrease. The index can vary within a range of 0 (absence of autoregulation) to 9 (best autoregulation). The best fit of the measured curve is the ARI value. Initially developed for the leg-cuff test, this approach has also been applicable to other methods and has therefore become widely used. The alternative autoregulatory slope index, evaluating the steepness of the slope of the CA response, shows a good correlation with the ARI.

The rate of recovery (RoR) has been defined, evaluating CA efficiency by analyzing the recovery time of the CBFV after an ABP-lowering stimulus [3]:

$$RoR = \frac{\frac{\triangle CVRi}{\triangle T}}{\triangle ABP}\ [CBFV/s].$$

Another way to evaluate CA in the time domain is the correlation coefficient (Mx) (Czosnyka et al. [12]), or the Pearson's correlation coefficient between ABP and the CBFV.

Evaluation of the frequency domain is performed using transfer function analysis. The relationship between ABP oscillations and CBF oscillations is analyzed. In other words, CA is quantified by considering the changes between the input signal ABP and the output CBF [10]. Three parameters are assessed: gain (or amplitude), phase shift, and coherence.

Efficient CA dampens the gain. Therefore, a low gain reflects intact CA, whereas an increase in the gain indicates diminished efficacy of CA. With intact CA, phase-shift analysis shows a positive phase difference between ABP and CBF, whereas the phase shift tends to disappear with decreasing CA [13]. Translated to the time domain, a phase shift of zero (no time delay between oscillations of ABP and the CBFV) reflects an absence of CA [10]. The linearity of the relationship between ABP and CBF can be described as coherence: a high coherence suggests a linear relationship, whereas coherence approaching zero indicates no linear relationship.

Studies in Humans

CA has been evaluated in several clinical conditions, especially in ICU situations. In patients with traumatic brain injury (TBI), CA was variably impaired within the first 2 weeks after head injury. Elevated ICP was an important factor associated with this impairment. Impaired CA was found to be an independent predictor of fatal outcome in TBI (see review by Czosnyka) [14].

In patients with subarachnoidal hemorrhage (SAH), a negative THR was found, with peaks at days 0–3 and at days 7–14 (with a significant association with cerebral vasospasm in these patients) [15]. In another study, these findings were confirmed for patients with aneurysmal SAH, indicating that CA impairment preceded vasospasm, worsened on-going vasospasm, and was also associated with a low CPP [16]. In a study administering statins to SAH patients, CA improved in the pravastatin group, indicating a benefit for patients at risk of vasospasm-related ischemic complications [17].

While the phase characteristics of dCA were not generally impaired in patients with acute intracerebral hemorrhage, the gain indicated CA disturbances. However, these changes were not related to clinical factors or outcome [18].

The effect of positive end-expiratory pressure ventilation in patients with acute respiratory distress syndrome has shown impairment of CA in >50% of the patients. In another ICU study of patients with sepsis and associated delirium, a potential role of impaired CA in sepsis-associated delirium was discussed. Impaired CA in a case of severe acute encephalitis has also been reported.

One major area of interest has been patients with acute ischemic stroke. A comprehensive review by Aries et al., summarizing 23 studies (16 on acute stroke and 7 on chronic stroke), has been published [19]. Three aspects were discussed: (1) Does CA impairment occur and why? CA impairment was found and seems to be related to endothelial and smooth muscle dysfunction of the vessels after ischemia. (2) How extensive is the impairment? CA was impaired not only in larger infarction but also in patients with lacunar stroke. As a second aspect, CA was impaired in both hemispheres and not restricted to the symptomatic side. However, it remains unclear if the disturbed CA in lacunar infarction is a result of chronic small-vessel disease in such patients or due to the acute infarction since longitudinal studies are missing. One small study has confirmed bihemispheric CA impairment in acute ischemic stroke, with a slightly more pronounced but not significantly different impairment in cortical stroke compared with subcortical stroke. (3) What is the time course? Studies with follow-up investigations showed increasing CA impairment during the first few days, persisting after 2 weeks in patients with larger stroke, whereas in patients with minor stroke, impairment was resolved after 2 weeks. Recovery phases lasting 3 months have been reported. In chronic stroke patients, arterial hypertension might play a role when CA impairment persists in the chronic phase after stroke since impaired CA in patients with malignant hypertension was reported. In patients with microangiopathy, impaired CA was found and significantly associated with the severity of chronic white matter lesions. Besides CA impairment in chronic hypertension, a shift of CA limits toward higher ABP levels has been found. This seems meaningful since the brain might be better protected against hypertension. However, the brain might be more vulnerable to hypoperfusion in situations of systemic hypotension. Recently, some authors hypothesized that pharmacological lowering of BP in older patients with hypertension might alter CA and therefore cause cognitive impairment.

CA assessment has been performed to characterize the hemodynamic severity of internal carotid artery (ICA) stenosis and the entailed risk for ischemic stroke. Factors such as the presence of collateral pathways are important, but intact CA compensating for reduced CPP by arteriolar dilatation might play a role (see reviews by Diehl et al. and Reinhard et al.) [20, 21]. In general, reduced CA has been found for an affected vessel compared with the contralateral side if the stenosis is at least 70%. A higher risk of stroke on the affected side compared with the unaffected side has been found, although it remains a topic of debate if disturbed CA by itself represents an independent risk factor for further strokes (for further detail, see review by Schytz et al.) [22]. CA has also been assessed in patients undergoing carotid surgery, showing a (partial) restoration of CA function after the intervention [23–25]. Studies on patients with severe middle cerebral artery (MCA) stenosis have shown impaired CA on the affected side. Decreased CA has also been shown in patients with bilateral severe ICA stenosis/occlusion. In contrast, in patients with mainly moderate posterior cerebral artery (PCA) stenosis, no significantly altered CA was found, potentially due to the lower grade of stenosis.

Studies in patients with *vasovagal syncope* mostly demonstrated impaired CA, showing a paradoxical cerebral vasoconstriction preceding the syncope. The discussion has been controversial since initially, this was interpreted as a paradoxical response to low systemic ABP. However, in a further study, cerebral vasoconstriction preceded the systemic ABP lowering, indicating an independent mechanism of vasoconstriction. The autonomic nerve system seems to play an important role. Overall, the detailed pathophysiology remains unclear (see review by Panerai) [2]. Dysregulated CA has also been described in patients with carotid sinus syndrome and in a patient suffering from eclampsia.

Since CA is severely impaired in mouse models of Alzheimer's disease (AD), it has been hypothesized that disturbed CA might play a role in the development of AD (e.g. by failing to protect the brain against ABP fluctuations and therefore favoring transient hypo- or hyperperfusion). However, recent preliminary studies in humans could not confirm major CA disturbances [26].

Cerebral Vasomotor Reactivity

Definition

Cerebral vasomotor reactivity (VMR) (synonym: cerebral vasoreactivity or CO_2 vasoreactivity) reflects the adaptation of the CBF to the arterial CO_2 pressure and the respective pH of the brain tissue. The cerebral vessels, especially on the level of small arterioles, are extremely sensitive to the vasodilatative effect of elevated arterial $PaCO_2$ concentrations (entailing higher velocities in TCD measurements), and therefore, VMR is considered as a surrogate of the function of the cerebral microcirculation and is indirectly useful to assess CA. VMR is defined as the 'ratio of percentage changes in CBFV to changes in $PaCO_2$' [27]:

$$VMR = \frac{100 \times \left(CBFVhyper - CBFVnorm\right)}{CBFVnorm \times \left(PCO_2 hyper - PCO_2 norm\right)} \left[\%/mm\ Hg\right].$$

Normal values for VMR have been reported to be about 5%/mm Hg (lower limit of 2%/mm Hg). Depending on the method (e.g. without a direct CO_2 stimulus), VMR might also be calculated as:

$$VMR = \frac{100 \times \left(CBFVhyper - CBFVnorm\right)}{CBFVnorm} \left[\%\right].$$

Normal values have been reported to be around 40% (lower limit of around 15%).

Animal Studies

No relevant fTCD animal studies providing additional information on VMR can be cited or overlap with the preceding chapter.

Several methods to measure VMR have been described. They are based either on the reaction to a CO_2 stimulus or on the application of another (e.g. pharmacological) vasodilatative stimulus.

To assess the breath-holding index (BHI) [28], the CBFV is measured for 1 min at baseline, followed by an apnea phase (breath holding). The baseline CBFV (CBFV rest) and the maximal CBFV during/after apnea (CBFV apnea) are recorded. The increase in the CBFV during the apnea interval (T apnea) is calculated as:

$$\text{BHI} = 100 \times \frac{\text{CBFVapnea} - \text{CBFVrest}}{\text{CBFVrest} \times \text{Tapnea}} \; [\%/s].$$

The BHI is free of any CO_2^- or pharmacological administration, making it useful as a screening tool. As a weakness, it requires cooperation of the patient and might be biased by a Valsalva maneuver during apnea. The achieved pCO_2 remains unknown.

The hyperventilation-apnea test consists of 30 s of hyperventilation followed by an apnea phase. The highest and lowest CBFV values are recorded. The same disadvantages as mentioned for the previous method persist.

Methods using CO_2 inhalation require more sophisticated technical settings. Two different approaches have been described:

The VMR range method (Ringelstein et al. [29]) plots relative CBFVs (the velocities under different CO_2 conditions relative to the velocity under room air conditions, the latter being defined as 100%) against corresponding end-tidal CO_2 concentrations. A tangent hyperbolic (s-shaped) function is fitted, resulting in 2 asymptotes, which represent the upper and lower limits of the VMR range.

The VMR slope method (Markwalder et al. [30]) uses 5 different conditions of CO_2 concentrations (normal air, mild and low hypocapnia, and inhalation of air with 7 or 5% CO_2) to plot the MCA velocity (VMCA) against the end-tidal PCO_2 as an exponential function curve. Recording is performed for 3–5 min after the steady PCO_2 concentration has been reached.

$$\text{VMR} = \frac{\text{dVMCA/VMCA}}{\text{dPCO}_2}.$$

Besides the more complex setting as a disadvantage, increasing CO_2 levels may induce the disagreeable sensation of asphyxia during CO_2 inhalation.

As a pharmacological approach, acetazolamide has high vasodilatative potency by blocking the carboanhydrase enzyme in erythrocytes and therefore inducing arterial acidosis and hypercapnia. During the acetazolamide test [31], the patient lays down, and the CBFV is recorded at baseline for 5 min, followed by an intravenous injection of 500–1,000 mg acetazolamide over approximately 1 min. After 1 min, a CBFV increase, which lasts about 15–20 min, can be observed.

The test is simpler than CO_2 application, and the patient does not need to cooperate; therefore, the test is widely used. However, compared with CO_2 application methods, it seems less accurate and less reproducible. Moreover, acetazolamide injection might induce counterproductive hyperventilation (partly neutralizing the vasodilative effect of the drug) and might have undesirable side effects, such as arterial hypertension, headache, nausea, and perioral dysesthesia.

Studies in Humans

Some overlaps between VMR and CA studies exist; some studies might have been reported in the previous chapter. In patients with ischemic stroke or ICA occlusive disease, patients with ICA occlusion demonstrated a significantly higher risk of ipsilateral ischemic events during follow-up in the subgroup with disturbed VMR [32–34]. However, in a recent study of patients with symptomatic ICA occlusion, disturbed VMR was not a significant risk factor for stroke recurrence [35]. In patients with asymptomatic ICA stenosis of at least 70%, the ipsilateral event rate in the subgroups with reduced VMR was significantly higher [34, 36, 37]. Some authors concluded that reduced VMR was an independent predictor of stroke [34]. Patients with ICA stenosis <70% showed no significant impairment [38, 39]. In a population with transient ischemic attack/minor stroke, a relationship between hypertension and cholesterol levels and CO_2 reactivity was found.

An improvement of VMR after medical treatment with statins as well as after rehabilitation with aerobic exercise has been reported in hemiparetic stroke survivors.

A few studies have investigated patients with cerebral microangiopathy and have found reduced VMR, reflecting a potential role for the small vessels in VMR [40].

In patients with TBI, testing VMR requires more precautions since the ICP might be unstable and since hypercapnia could entail a reduction of the CPP. Impairment of VMR in these patients has been reported and has shown some association with the clinical outcome [29, 41]. Impaired VMR has also been found in patients with sleep apnea [42] or hypertension [43].

Neurovascular Coupling

Definition

The response of cerebral hemodynamics to neuronal activity and elevated metabolism, leading to functional hyperemia, is based on NVC, reflecting interactions of the 'neurovascular unit' (formed by neurons, astrocytes, and vascular cells) [44]. Changes in the CBFV are likely to reflect changes in the cerebral blood volume resulting from neuronal activity in the supplied field.

Animal Studies

A mouse study using laser-Doppler flowmetry provided some evidence for impaired NVC due to arterial hypertension [45]. The increase in CBF after somatosensory stimulation in transgenic mice with overexpression of β-amyloid precursor protein is significantly reduced compared with the increase in healthy controls. Disturbed mechanisms of energy supply and demand caused by β-amyloid precursor protein depositions have been incriminated. Further evidence of cerebrovascular dysfunction due to β-amyloid depositions in cerebral amyloid angiopathy (CAA) has been provided [46]. For more details on NVC in AD, see the review by Nicolakakis and Hamel [47].

Overall, one needs to keep in mind that most of the animal studies were performed under anesthesia, which might influence NVC, and that the direct translation of these findings to human conditions has to be done with precaution.

Methods in Humans

In humans, the CBFV can be recorded in either the MCA or the PCA, preferably bilaterally since interhemispheric comparisons seem to be useful in most cases. For MCA recording, different stimuli have been used (e.g. motor, sensory, cognitive, or emotional stimulation), according to the aim of the study. For PCA recording, a visual stimulus is meaningful. Different techniques have been reported, distinguishing between flickering light; a checkerboard black/white pattern; or, as the most complex stimulus evoking the highest amplitudes of the CBFV, a rotating colored optokinetic drum. The most common analyzed parameter is the (relative) evoked flow (e.g. with visual stimulation):

$$\text{VEFR} = \frac{v_{max} - v_0}{v_0} \times 100, \left[\%\right]$$

(VEFR = visually evoked flow response; v_{max} = the maximum CBFV after stimulation; v_0 = the CBFV at rest).

Other parameters, such as the latency of the CBF increase and the steepness of the increasing or decreasing slope, can also be analyzed and might be of interest in specific contexts. Some studies have used complex mathematical equations to interpret the data.

Studies in Humans

Studies in Healthy Humans
The possibility to record the effects of NVC improved our understanding of specific brain functions, especially in the pre-fMRI era. fTCD studies have been useful to de-

scribe the brain's organization. Concerning topography, some of the results have been confirmed to be compatible with results in fMRI studies.

After first experiences with simple *visual stimuli* (the VEFR in the PCA) [48] and *motor tasks* (contralateral activation of the MCA), more complex settings with cognitive tasks have been a major issue. A basic finding in healthy subjects within different age groups undergoing visual stimulation suggested that NVC remains unaffected during normal aging [49].

A significantly higher evoked flow response in the left MCA has been reported as an indicator of language lateralization in the left hemisphere. This fTCD approach has been compared with the Wada test as the gold standard and has shown concordant results. For clinical practice, this method has been proposed for evaluating patients before they undergo brain surgery, e.g. patients with temporal lobe epilepsy surgery.

Other studies have investigated the evoked flow in the MCA with complex spatial tasks, evoking blood flow activation in the right MCA, as well as with memory tasks such as picture recognition, which also evoked right hemispheric activation [50]. Spatial orientation paradigms have been shown to be useful for detection of the nondominant hemisphere.

In a study on attention processes, no significant lateralization was found. Emotional processing seems to involve the right hemisphere since MCA recording during presentation of negative emotional content showed activation in the right MCA compared with presentation of non-emotional content.

With auditory stimulation, different activations could be recorded in response to noise (not lateralized), speech recognition (left hemispheric activation), melody perception (bihemispheric), or recognition (right hemispheric activation). A review of fTCD studies and psychophysical functions has been published by Duschek and Schandry [51].

A more recent approach was to investigate the nociceptive response in patients after heat stimulation. fTCD showed a corresponding CBF increase in the anterior cerebral artery and MCA. Therefore, fTCD might become a tool in pain research to further characterize nociceptive processing mechanisms [52].

Studies under Pathologic Conditions
Disruption of NVC has been postulated to occur in patients with arterial hypertension, ischemic stroke [53], or cerebrovascular diseases more generally. Some studies using fMRI or PET have confirmed these assumptions, although specific fTCD studies are scarce or lacking.

In a study on patients with ischemic stroke (not affecting the PCA territory), visual stimulation induced significantly lower responses in patients compared with healthy controls, confirming the hypothesis of disturbed NVC in such patients [54]. There was no difference between the subgroups of ischemic stroke due to large-artery intracranial stenosis compared with small-vessel disease.

In patients with CAA, an impaired VEFR after visual stimulation probably reflects pathologies of the distal resistance vessels in CAA [55].

Patients suffering from migraine have been investigated extensively, mostly using a visual stimulation paradigm. The results have been variable, with an either increased or decreased VEFR or with asymmetries in the VEFR [56], indicating a disturbed hemodynamic response [57].

In a small study on type I diabetes patients, fTCD was useful for detecting increased attenuation, probably reflecting endothelial dysfunction with increased wall rigidity as a precursor of atherosclerosis.

Impaired VEFRs have also been described in smokers. Disturbed responses remained after smoking cessation, possibly indicating structural changes of the vessels in these subjects [58].

fTCD has also been performed to get insight into functional processes during rehabilitation. A systematic review by Salinet et al. summarizes the heterogeneous results, with not only contralateral but also ipsilateral activation during motor or cognitive tasks [59].

Disturbed hemodynamic regulation and a lower VEFR have been found in patients with AD. After treatment with acetylcholine esterase inhibitors, vascular regulation improved significantly. It remains unclear if the disturbed vascular response in AD is due to a decreased demand for blood as a consequence of brain tissue pathology or if it primarily reflects a problem with the vessels, e.g. due to the deposition of amyloid in the vessel walls (amyloid angiopathy) or due to perivascular denervation because of the cholinotoxic properties of β-amyloid [47]. For a comprehensive overview of TCD in dementia, see the review by Keage et al. [60].

In a small study of patients with Parkinson's disease, a significant difference in the evoked CBF during presentation of a negative emotional task was found, matching the deficit in emotional processing in patients with Parkinson's disease.

In general, fTCD studies have mainly been used to evaluate and understand specific brain functions in healthy subjects and to characterize NVC in patients with migraine or cerebrovascular diseases. With the increasing availability of fMRI, the number of fTCD studies has decreased. However, the application of fTCD has been extended from patients with cerebrovascular diseases to patients with neurodegenerative diseases. In future studies, approaches combining the techniques of fTCD and fMRI might provide additional information [61].

References

1 Strebel S, Lam AM, Matta B, Mayberg TS, Aaslid R, Newell DW: Dynamic and static cerebral autoregulation during isoflurane, desflurane, and propofol anesthesia. Anesthesiology 1995;83:66–76.

2 Panerai RB: Transcranial Doppler for evaluation of cerebral autoregulation. Clin Auton Res 2009;19: 197–211.

3 Aaslid R, Lindegaard KF, Sorteberg W, Nornes H: Cerebral autoregulation dynamics in humans. Stroke 1989;20:45–52.

4 Aaslid R: Cerebral autoregulation and vasomotor reactivity. Front Neurol Neurosci 2006;21:216–228.

5 Giller CA: A bedside test for cerebral autoregulation using transcranial Doppler ultrasound. Acta Neurochir (Wien) 1991;108:7–14.

6 Tiecks FP, Douville C, Byrd S, Lam AM, Newell DW: Evaluation of impaired cerebral autoregulation by the Valsalva maneuver. Stroke 1996;27:1177–1182.

7 Lipsitz LA, Mukai S, Hamner J, Gagnon M, Babikian V: Dynamic regulation of middle cerebral artery blood flow velocity in aging and hypertension. Stroke 2000;31:1897–1903.

8 Sorond FA, Serrador JM, Jones RN, Shaffer ML, Lipsitz LA: The sit-to-stand technique for the measurement of dynamic cerebral autoregulation. Ultrasound Med Biol 2009;35:21–29.

9 Birch AA, Neil-Dwyer G, Murrills AJ: The repeatability of cerebral autoregulation assessment using sinusoidal lower body negative pressure. Physiol Meas 2002;23:73–83.

10 van Beek AH, Claassen JA, Rikkert MG, Jansen RW: Cerebral autoregulation: an overview of current concepts and methodology with special focus on the elderly. J Cereb Blood Flow Metab 2008;28:1071–1085.

11 Tiecks FP, Lam AM, Aaslid R, Newell DW: Comparison of static and dynamic cerebral autoregulation measurements. Stroke 1995;26:1014–1019.

12 Czosnyka M, Smielewski P, Kirkpatrick P, Menon DK, Pickard JD: Monitoring of cerebral autoregulation in head-injured patients. Stroke 1996;27:1829–1834.

13 Diehl RR, Linden D, Lucke D, Berlit P: Phase relationship between cerebral blood flow velocity and blood pressure. A clinical test of autoregulation. Stroke 1995;26:1801–1804.

14 Czosnyka M, Brady K, Reinhard M, Smielewski P, Steiner LA: Monitoring of cerebrovascular autoregulation: facts, myths, and missing links. Neurocrit Care 2009;10:373–386.

15 Ratsep T, Asser T: Cerebral hemodynamic impairment after aneurysmal subarachnoid hemorrhage as evaluated using transcranial Doppler ultrasonography: relationship to delayed cerebral ischemia and clinical outcome. J Neurosurg 2001;95:393–401.

16 Lang EW, Diehl RR, Mehdorn HM: Cerebral autoregulation testing after aneurysmal subarachnoid hemorrhage: the phase relationship between arterial blood pressure and cerebral blood flow velocity. Crit Care Med 2001;29:158–163.

17 Tseng MY, Czosnyka M, Richards H, Pickard JD, Kirkpatrick PJ: Effects of acute treatment with statins on cerebral autoregulation in patients after aneurysmal subarachnoid hemorrhage. Neurosurg Focus 2006;21:E10.

18 Oeinck M, Neunhoeffer F, Buttler KJ, Meckel S, Schmidt B, Czosnyka M, et al: Dynamic cerebral autoregulation in acute intracerebral hemorrhage. Stroke 2013;44:2722–2728.

19 Aries MJ, Elting JW, De Keyser J, Kremer BP, Vroomen PC: Cerebral autoregulation in stroke: a review of transcranial Doppler studies. Stroke 2010;41:2697–2704.

20 Diehl RR: Cerebral autoregulation studies in clinical practice. Eur J Ultrasound 2002;16:31–36.

21 Reinhard M, Gerds TA, Grabiak D, Zimmermann PR, Roth M, Guschlbauer B, et al: Cerebral dysautoregulation and the risk of ischemic events in occlusive carotid artery disease. J Neurol 2008;255:1182–1189.

22 Schytz HW, Hansson A, Phillip D, Selb J, Boas DA, Iversen HK, et al: Spontaneous low-frequency oscillations in cerebral vessels: applications in carotid artery disease and ischemic stroke. J Stroke Cerebrovasc Dis 2010;19:465–474.

23 Reinhard M, Roth M, Muller T, Guschlbauer B, Timmer J, Czosnyka M, et al: Effect of carotid endarterectomy or stenting on impairment of dynamic cerebral autoregulation. Stroke 2004;35:1381–1387.

24 Telman G, Kouperberg E, Nitecki S, Karram T, Schwarz HA, Sprecher E, et al: Cerebral hemodynamics in symptomatic and asymptomatic patients with severe unilateral carotid stenosis before and after carotid endarterectomy. Eur J Vasc Endovasc Surg 2006;32:375–378.

25 Mense L, Reimann M, Rudiger H, Gahn G, Reichmann H, Hentschel H, et al: Autonomic function and cerebral autoregulation in patients undergoing carotid endarterectomy. Circ J 2010;74:2139–2145.

26 Claassen JA, Zhang R: Cerebral autoregulation in Alzheimer's disease. J Cereb Blood Flow Metab 2011;31:1572–1577.

27 Purkayastha S, Sorond F: Transcranial Doppler ultrasound: technique and application. Semin Neurol 2012;32:411–420.

28 Markus HS, Harrison MJ: Estimation of cerebrovascular reactivity using transcranial Doppler, including the use of breath-holding as the vasodilatory stimulus. Stroke 1992;23:668–673.

29 Ringelstein EB, Sievers C, Ecker S, Schneider PA, Otis SM: Noninvasive assessment of CO2-induced cerebral vasomotor response in normal individuals and patients with internal carotid artery occlusions. Stroke 1988;19:963–969.

30 Markwalder TM, Grolimund P, Seiler RW, Roth F, Aaslid R: Dependency of blood flow velocity in the middle cerebral artery on end-tidal carbon dioxide partial pressure – a transcranial ultrasound Doppler study. J Cereb Blood Flow Metab 1984;4:368–372.

31 Dahl A, Russell D, Rootwelt K, Nyberg-Hansen R, Kerty E: Cerebral vasoreactivity assessed with transcranial Doppler and regional cerebral blood flow measurements. Dose, serum concentration, and time course of the response to acetazolamide. Stroke 1995;26:2302–2306.

32 Kleiser B, Widder B: Course of carotid artery occlusions with impaired cerebrovascular reactivity. Stroke 1992;23:171–174.

33 Vernieri F, Pasqualetti P, Matteis M, Passarelli F, Troisi E, Rossini PM, et al: Effect of collateral blood flow and cerebral vasomotor reactivity on the outcome of carotid artery occlusion. Stroke 2001;32:1552–1558.

34 Markus H, Cullinane M: Severely impaired cerebrovascular reactivity predicts stroke and TIA risk in patients with carotid artery stenosis and occlusion. Brain 2001;124:457–467.

35 Jolink WM, Heinen R, Persoon S, van der Zwan A, Kappelle LJ, Klijn CJ: Transcranial Doppler ultrasonography CO2 reactivity does not predict recurrent ischaemic stroke in patients with symptomatic carotid artery occlusion. Cerebrovasc Dis 2014;37:30–37.

36 Gur AY, Bova I, Bornstein NM: Is impaired cerebral vasomotor reactivity a predictive factor of stroke in asymptomatic patients? Stroke 1996;27:2188–2190.

37 Silvestrini M, Vernieri F, Pasqualetti P, Matteis M, Passarelli F, Troisi E, et al: Impaired cerebral vasoreactivity and risk of stroke in patients with asymptomatic carotid artery stenosis. JAMA 2000;283:2122–2127.

38 Naylor AR, Merrick MV, Gillespie I, Sandercock PA, Warlow CP, Cull RE, et al: Prevalence of impaired cerebrovascular reserve in patients with symptomatic carotid artery disease. Br J Surg 1994;81:45–48.

39 Pericot I, Molina C, Alvarez-Sabin J, Codina A: [The influence of the arterial pressure in the study of cerebrovascular reactivity in carotid obstructions]. Rev Neurol 2000;31:1015–1018.

40 Bakker SL, de Leeuw FE, de Groot JC, Hofman A, Koudstaal PJ, Breteler MM: Cerebral vasomotor reactivity and cerebral white matter lesions in the elderly. Neurology 1999;52:578–583.

41 Lee JH, Kelly DF, Oertel M, McArthur DL, Glenn TC, Vespa P, et al: Carbon dioxide reactivity, pressure autoregulation, and metabolic suppression reactivity after head injury: a transcranial Doppler study. J Neurosurg 2001;95:222–232.

42 Reichmuth KJ, Dopp JM, Barczi SR, Skatrud JB, Wojdyla P, Hayes D Jr, et al: Impaired vascular regulation in patients with obstructive sleep apnea: effects of continuous positive airway pressure treatment. Am J Respir Crit Care Med 2009;180:1143–1150.

43 Serrador JM, Sorond FA, Vyas M, Gagnon M, Iloputaife ID, Lipsitz LA: Cerebral pressure-flow relations in hypertensive elderly humans: transfer gain in different frequency domains. J Appl Physiol 2005;98:151–159.

44 Iadecola C: Neurovascular regulation in the normal brain and in Alzheimer's disease. Nat Rev Neurosci 2004;5:347–360.

45 Kazama K, Wang G, Frys K, Anrather J, Iadecola C: Angiotensin II attenuates functional hyperemia in the mouse somatosensory cortex. Am J Physiol Heart Circ Physiol 2003;285:H1890–H1899.

46 Shin HK, Jones PB, Garcia-Alloza M, Borrelli L, Greenberg SM, Bacskai BJ, et al: Age-dependent cerebrovascular dysfunction in a transgenic mouse model of cerebral amyloid angiopathy. Brain 2007;130:2310–2319.

47 Nicolakakis N, Hamel E: Neurovascular function in Alzheimer's disease patients and experimental models. J Cereb Blood Flow Metab 2011;31:1354–1370.

48 Aaslid R: Visually evoked dynamic blood flow response of the human cerebral circulation. Stroke 1987;18:771–775.

49 Rosengarten B, Aldinger C, Spiller A, Kaps M: Neurovascular coupling remains unaffected during normal aging. J Neuroimaging 2003;13:43–47.

50 Klingelhofer J, Matzander G, Sander D, Schwarze J, Boecker H, Bischoff C: Assessment of functional hemispheric asymmetry by bilateral simultaneous cerebral blood flow velocity monitoring. J Cereb Blood Flow Metab 1997;17:577–585.

51 Duschek S, Schandry R: Functional transcranial Doppler sonography as a tool in psychophysiological research. Psychophysiology 2003;40:436–454.

52 Duschek S, Hellmann N, Merzoug K, Reyes del Paso GA, Werner NS: Cerebral blood flow dynamics during pain processing investigated by functional transcranial Doppler sonography. Pain Med 2012;13:419–426.

53 Girouard H, Iadecola C: Neurovascular coupling in the normal brain and in hypertension, stroke, and Alzheimer disease. J Appl Physiol 2006;100:328–335.

54 Lin WH, Hao Q, Rosengarten B, Leung WH, Wong KS: Impaired neurovascular coupling in ischaemic stroke patients with large or small vessel disease. Eur J Neurol 2011;18:731–736.

55 Smith EE, Vijayappa M, Lima F, Delgado P, Wendell L, Rosand J, et al: Impaired visual evoked flow velocity response in cerebral amyloid angiopathy. Neurology 2008;71:1424–1430.

56 Wolf ME, Jager T, Bazner H, Hennerici M: Changes in functional vasomotor reactivity in migraine with aura. Cephalalgia 2009;29:1156–1164.

57 Nowak A, Kacinski M: Transcranial Doppler evaluation in migraineurs. Neurol Neurochir Pol 2009;43:162–172.

58 Boms N, Yonai Y, Molnar S, Rosengarten B, Bornstein NM, Csiba L, et al: Effect of smoking cessation on visually evoked cerebral blood flow response in healthy volunteers. J Vasc Res 2010;47:214–220.

59 Salinet AS, Haunton VJ, Panerai RB, Robinson TG: A systematic review of cerebral hemodynamic responses to neural activation following stroke. J Neurol 2013;260:2715–2721.

60 Keage HA, Churches OF, Kohler M, Pomeroy D, Luppino R, Bartolo ML, et al: Cerebrovascular function in aging and dementia: a systematic review of transcranial Doppler studies. Dement Geriatr Cogn Dis Extra 2012;2:258–270.

61 Griebe M, Flux F, Wolf ME, Hennerici MG, Szabo K: Multimodal assessment of optokinetic visual stimulation response in migraine with aura. Headache 2014;54:131–141.

Dr. Marc E. Wolf
Department of Neurology
Universitätsmedizin Mannheim, University of Heidelberg
Theodor-Kutzer-Ufer 1–3, DE–68167 Mannheim (Germany)
E-Mail wolf@neuro.ma.uni-heidelberg.de

Alonso A, Hennerici MG, Meairs S (eds): Translational Neurosonology.
Front Neurol Neurosci. Basel, Karger, 2015, vol 36, pp 57–70 (DOI: 10.1159/000366237)

Intracranial Perfusion Imaging with Ultrasound

Stephen Meairs · Rolf Kern

Department of Neurology, Universitätsmedizin Mannheim, University of Heidelberg, Mannheim, Germany

Abstract

In the last several years, great progress has been made in ultrasound perfusion imaging of the brain. Different approaches have been assessed and shown to be capable of the early detection of cerebral perfusion deficits in stroke patients. Real-time low-mechanical index imaging simplifies the acquisition of perfusion parameters and alleviates many of the previous imaging problems related to shadowing, uniplanar analysis, and temporal resolution. With the advent of this new, highly sensitive contrast-specific imaging technique, new possibilities of the real-time visualization of brain infarctions and cerebral hemorrhages have emerged. This review will detail the methodology of ultrasound perfusion imaging, discuss aspects of its safety and present the emerging clinical applications of brain perfusion assessment with ultrasound in acute stroke patients.

Background

There is evidence from several experimental and clinical studies that ultrasound can be used to depict blood flow in the microcirculation of the brain [1–5]. In contrast to other techniques for the assessment of cerebral blood flow (e.g. single photon emission computed tomography), ultrasound is a relatively simple, affordable and largely widespread bedside imaging technique. The introduction of new ultrasound contrast agents (UCAs) and the development of contrast-specific imaging modalities have opened new possibilities for the application of ultrasound, e.g. in stroke patients.

In clinical settings, intracranial perfusion imaging with ultrasound has been limited to semi-quantitative studies for the characterization of perfusion abnormalities [6–8]. This is in contrast to ultrasound applications in other organs, such as the heart [9] and kidney [10, 11] and the skeletal muscle [12], where the in vivo measurements of tissue blood flow have been obtained by the implementation of microbubble replenishment kinetics [9].

The main limitations of this method have been the attenuation of the ultrasound by the human skull and the inter-individual variances in skull thickness [13, 14]. Because of the strong absorption of acoustic signals by the skull, the imaging of echo signals from microbubbles found in the brain microcirculation requires a high acoustic power. However, because UCAs are very fragile, this high power causes them to burst during insonation [15]. This results in a relevant decrease in the temporal resolution of the ultrasound brain perfusion imaging and, thus, of the sensitivity of this method to detect small differences in cerebral perfusion between different regions of interest (ROIs) [16]. Recent technological advances in ultrasound equipment showing improved sensitivity for the detection of microbubbles in cerebral microcirculation now enable real-time ultrasound brain perfusion imaging through the acoustic bone window in humans [17, 18].

Methodology of Intracranial Perfusion Imaging with Ultrasound

High-Mechanical Index Ultrasound Imaging
Most studies on the assessment of cerebral perfusion after UCA injection have applied high-mechanical index (MI) ultrasound imaging, regardless of the technique used for contrast-specific imaging. The MI, which was originally defined to predict the onset of cavitation in fluids, is a measure of acoustic output and also describes the likelihood of microbubble disruption. Until recently, there have been no alternatives to high-MI imaging because lower acoustic outputs have been unable to detect microbubbles in the brain. Therefore, because the bubbles are destroyed in the microcirculation during high-MI imaging, a triggered pulsing sequence is implemented to allow for the replenishment of new bubbles in the ultrasound scan plane. Accordingly, most early studies of cerebral perfusion have been performed with triggered harmonic gray-scale imaging techniques (conventional, power modulation or pulse-inversion), analyzing the bolus kinetics in healthy subjects to determine the best method for the detection of UCAs in the cerebral microcirculation [1, 2, 7, 19–29]. In some experiments, fundamental color duplex technologies based on the power Doppler mode and contrast agent destruction have been used (contrast burst imaging and time variance imaging).

Low-Mechanical Index Ultrasound Imaging
Low-MI real-time perfusion techniques allow for the detection of UCAs in the cerebral microcirculation with little or no bubble destruction compared to high MI-imaging (fig. 1). Because of the minimal contrast agent bubble destruction, a high frame rate can be applied, which leads to a better time resolution of bolus kinetics (fig. 2). The low-MI imaging of contrast agents also avoids the shadowing effect,

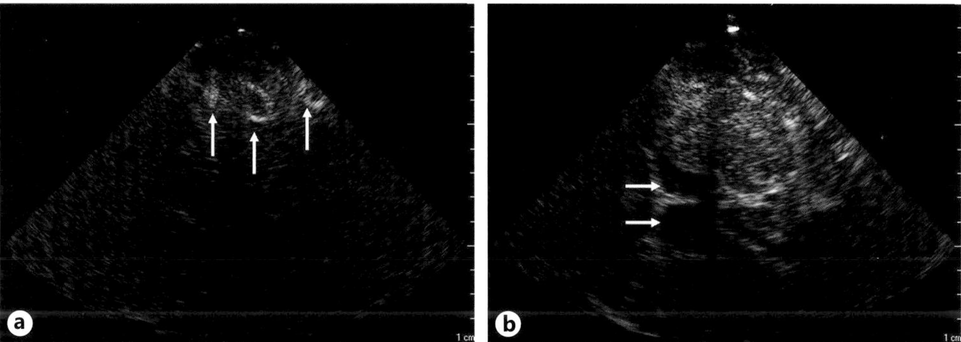

Fig. 1. Real-time display of brain perfusion with low-MI perfusion imaging of the brain on a Philips IU22 platform using a 1–5-MHz dynamic pulsed-array transducer. **a** The arrival of the contrast agent SonoVue™ is first observed in the M3 segments of the middle cerebral artery (arrows). **b** Thereafter, the contrast agent is delivered to the capillaries, which are then depicted by contrast-specific ultrasound as a homogenous contrast enhancement in the brain tissue. For anatomical reference, the arrows show the well-delineated frontal horns of the lateral ventricles.

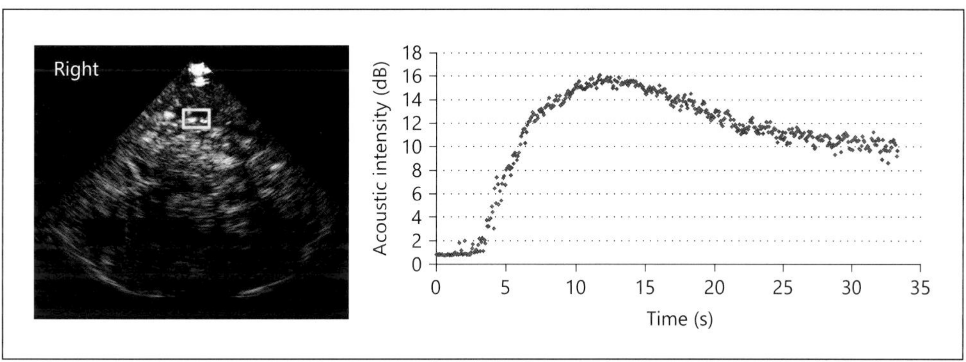

Fig. 2. Real-time acoustic intensity curve of the contrast agent SonoVue™ after bolus injection on a Philips IU22 platform using a 1–5-MHz dynamic pulsed-array transducer. A very low MI of 0.017 was used, which was then attenuated by approximately 90% by the skull bone before entering the brain. A region of interest is depicted in the upper image where the mean acoustic intensity will be measured.

which is a significant problem associated with high-MI imaging. Because of the high acoustic intensities that are emitted by the bursting bubbles, the bubbles that are 'behind' the emitting bubbles (further away from the ultrasound transducer) are 'shadowed' and are thus obscured from data analysis. The problem of shadowing is basically eliminated with low-MI imaging because the bubbles are not destroyed at such low acoustic pressures. Moreover, this technique has the potential for the repeated and multi-planar real-time measurement of brain perfusion [30]. This is a significant advantage over high-MI imaging protocols, which are confined to a sin-

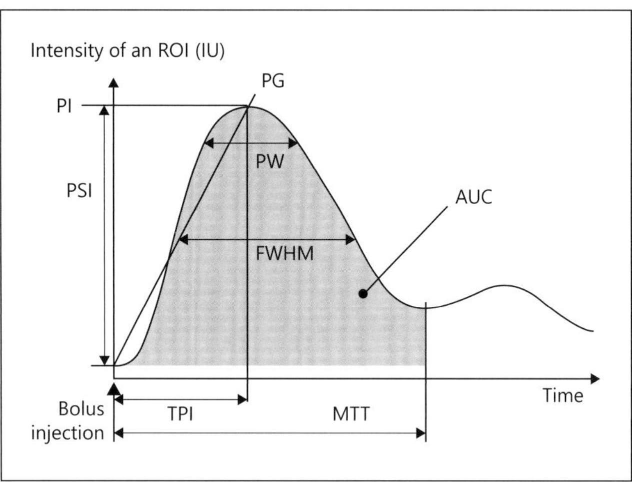

Fig. 3. Schematic representation of the different parameters of the time-intensity curve available for the perfusion assessment. ROI = Region of interest; IU = intensity units (linear scale); PI = peak intensity; PG = positive gradient; PSI = peak signal increase; PW = peak width; FWHM = full width at half of the maximum intensity; AUC = area under the curve; MTT = mean transit time.

gle image plane and are therefore limited in their assessments of the extents of brain infarction and low-perfusion states. The disadvantage of this low-MI technique, however, is the limited investigation depth due to the low MI used. Successful perfusion imaging of the contralateral hemisphere has not yet been demonstrated with this technique.

Microbubble Bolus Kinetics

After UCA bolus injection, time intensity curves with contrast wash-in and wash-out phases can be generated using contrast-specific imaging and further analysis *(bolus kinetics)*. Different parameters of these curves can be extracted (fig. 3), such as the time-to-peak intensity (TPI), the peak intensity (PI), the mean transit time, the peak width (full width at 90% of the maximum intensity) and the full width at half of the maximum intensity, the area under the curve, the positive gradient (defined as PI/TPI), and the peak signal increase. These parameters can then be displayed as parametric images [31]. Several studies have shown that such parameters may be suitable for the assessment of brain perfusion, particularly the analysis of local time-intensity curves in pre-specified ROIs [4] or the visual interpretation of parametric images [8, 31–34]. MRI and PET studies of acute stroke patients have demonstrated the diagnostic value of TPI maps for the differentiation between unaffected parenchyma, penumbra, and the ischemic core area [35]. Similar results have been achieved with ultrasound perfusion techniques.

Microbubble Destruction Kinetics

As an alternative imaging modality, *destruction kinetics* involves the destruction of contrast agent microbubbles at a constant frame rate using a high MI. After contrast bolus injection, the microbubbles are destroyed using a series of high-energy pulses. The local perfusion status is analyzed in selected ROIs by destruction curves and

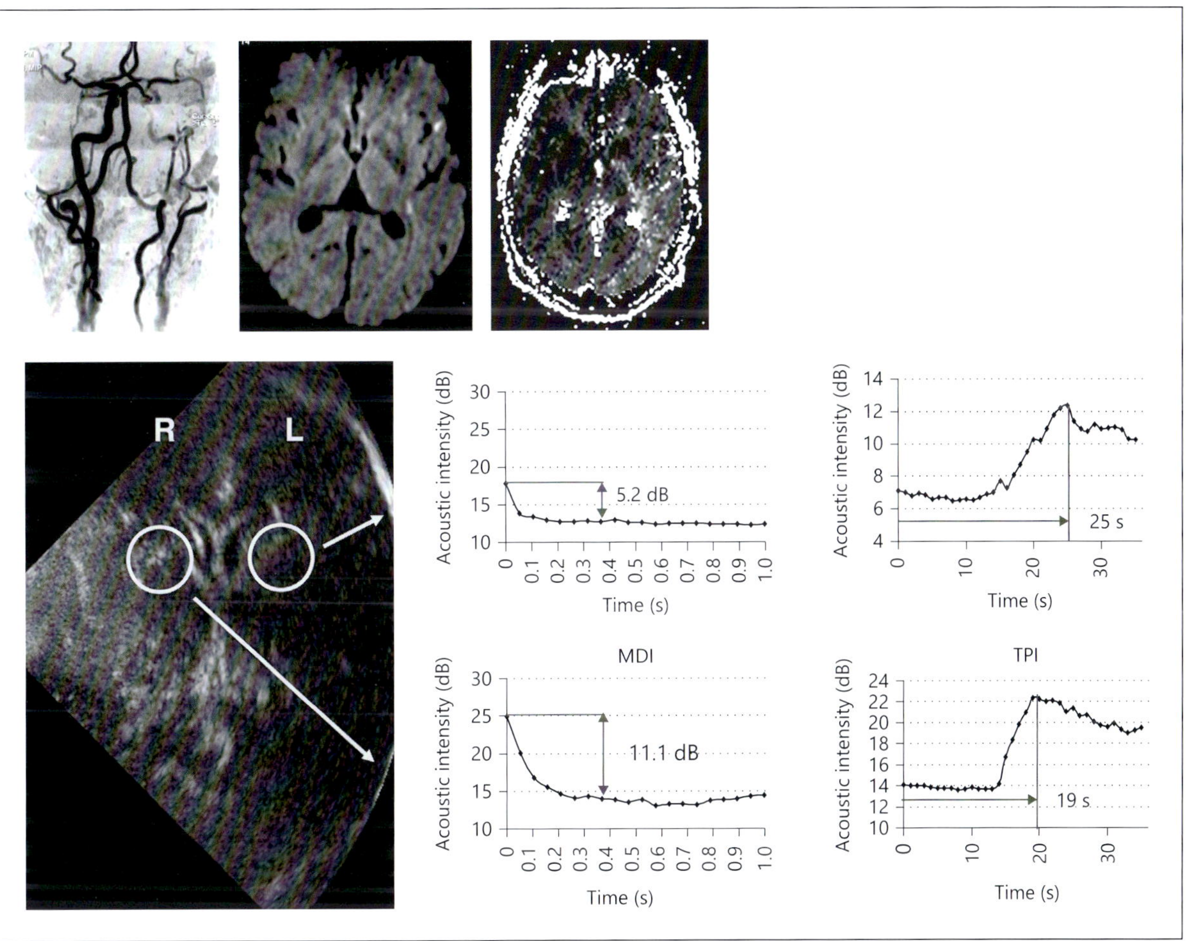

Fig. 4. Investigation of symptomatic high-grade left carotid stenosis with time-to-peak intensity (TPI) and microbubble-destruction imaging (MDI) using SonoVue™. The upper MRI images demonstrate the high-grade stenosis with MR angiography (left), left-hemispheric DWI lesions (middle) and the perfusion deficit in the left hemisphere as shown by perfusion-weighted imaging (right). For TPI, triggered imaging was used (frame rate of 1 Hz) to measure the time-to-maximum acoustic intensity. For the destruction imaging, repetitive sequences of high-energy pulses at a high frame rate (14 Hz), resulting in complete microbubble destruction, were applied. The analysis of TPI and MDI were undertaken in both hemispheres in the territory of the middle cerebral arteries (circles). Note both the prolonged TPI and the decreased destruction intensities in the left hemisphere.

acoustic intensity differences obtained before and after microbubble destruction [6, 36]. There are three mathematical models for analyzing the diminution curve; a linear, a simple exponential, and a complex exponential (contrast burst depletion imaging) model [22, 23, 36, 37]. Figure 4 provides an example of using microbubble destruction imaging to assess cerebral perfusion in a patient with a high-grade carotid stenosis.

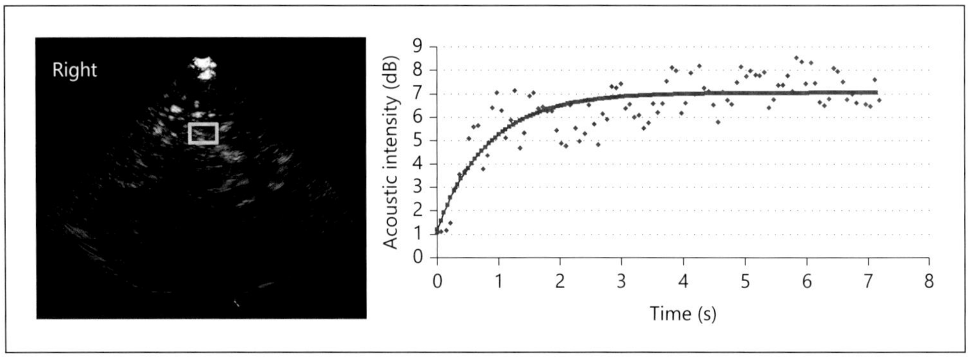

Fig. 5. Real-time acoustic intensity curve of the contrast agent SonoVue™, demonstrating refill following bubble destruction with transient high-MI imaging. Mean acoustic intensity is measured in the rectangular region of interest.

Microbubble Replenishment Kinetics

Another method to measure tissue perfusion with ultrasound is 'refill' or *replenishment kinetics*, which was first used by Wei and coworkers in myocardial tissue [9]. If a constant concentration of contrast agent is delivered to brain tissue using a constant UCA infusion rate, then after destruction with high-MI ultrasound, new microbubbles will enter this field with a certain velocity, which will travel a determined distance and fill a certain tissue volume depending on the blood velocity. The intensity of the echo response signal is directly related to the contrast agent concentration in the tissue, and therefore, the blood flow assessment is based on monitoring the intensity of the echo response signal of the insonated volume after the bubble destruction. Low-MI ultrasound imaging can be used to monitor microbubble replenishment in real time (fig. 5) following the application of destruction pulses at a high MI. The replenishment can be demonstrated by the exponential curve fit to $y = A(1-e^{\beta t})$, where A represents the plateau of the acoustic intensity, and β is the slope factor of the exponential curve [38]. These parameters are related to cerebral blood flow; blood flow velocity is directly related to the rate constant β, the fractional vascular volume is related to the plateau echo enhancement A, and the product of both $(A \times \beta)$ is associated with blood flow. Using the flash-replenishment mode of low-MI contrast agent imaging, refill kinetics can be analyzed very quickly (<5 s scanning time) compared to the high-MI approach (approximately 3 min scanning time).

Replenishment kinetics have been employed successfully to measure cerebral perfusion in an animal model of trepanated dogs, showing a good correlation with cerebral blood flow [39]. Different from the situation in humans, however, the brain was scanned through a craniotomy in the parietal bone, thus allowing for bubble destruction with high MI followed by real-time low-MI imaging of the replenishment in the dog brain. One early attempt to use refill kinetics in humans was undertaken by Seidel and coworkers in a group of healthy volunteers [24]. This study, however, was limited by triggered imaging sequences and low temporal resolution because the refill phase could only be imaged with high MI through the temporal bone window.

It remains unclear which kinetics or which parameter is the most valuable for the analysis of brain perfusion in healthy subjects. Theoretically, time-dependent parameters, such as the TPI *(bolus kinetics)*, the half-life perfusion coefficient *(diminution kinetics)*, or the β-value *(replenishment kinetics)* should be more useful than amplitude-dependent parameters because the latter also depend on insonation depth and the attenuation of the skull bone.

Safety of Ultrasound Perfusion Imaging

The commercially available UCAs Levovist™, Optison™, and SonoVue™ have been shown to have contrast enhancing properties in human brain perfusion imaging. No severe adverse events have been documented in numerous volunteer studies published on brain perfusion analyses using these contrast agents, which have included hundreds of patients.

One study investigated the integrity of the blood-brain barrier (BBB) in humans after the bubble destruction of Levovist™ and Optison™ with transcranial color-coded sonography [19]. MRI examinations with gadolinium (Gd-MRI) were performed during both the early and late phases after insonation. The ultrasound transmission power levels were kept within diagnostic limits and resembled the standard settings used in brain perfusion studies. Using a triple dose of gadolinium to increase sensitivity and considering the potential time dependence of the BBB changes, the authors showed that the insonation of Levovist™ and Optison™ did not lead to any detectable differences in the T1 signal intensities in the two defined brain regions by Gd-MRI. Moreover, they found no signs of focal signal enhancement or of focal brain damage. In another study of patients with small-vessel disease and intact BBBs, standard contrast-enhanced ultrasound perfusion imaging did not lead to MRI-detectable BBB changes [40]. These studies provide further evidence of the safety of UCAs and of the exposure levels of the current ultrasonic equipment used for transcranial investigations. The results are reassuring but not totally conclusive in terms of ultrasound safety because, hypothetically, the more subtle effects of ultrasounds and microbubbles on the BBB might be missed by Gd-MRI.

Experimental data also have suggested that microbubbles and ultrasounds have no deleterious effects on acute stroke. In one study [41], transcranial ultrasound was applied after the experimental induction of intracranial hemorrhages to rat brains for 30 min during a continuous intravenous infusion of SonoVue™. The results showed no significant effects of the ultrasound or the microbubbles on hemorrhage size, on the extent of brain edema, or on the rate of apoptosis. In another study, ultrasound and microbubbles (SonoVue™) were applied to a middle cerebral artery (MCA) occlusion model in rats to evaluate their possible effects on brain infarct volume, apoptosis, IL-6 and TNF-alpha levels, and the disruption of the BBB [42]. Interestingly, the results showed that infarct volume was significantly reduced in the microbubble and ultrasound groups compared to the control animals. The levels of IL-6 and TNF-alpha as markers of tissue damage were not significantly different. In the trypan blue-treated animals, no additional BBB disruptions were observed. Likewise, there was no increase in apoptotic cell death outside of the infarction area in the animals treated with the microbubbles and ultrasound. These results support the notion that ultrasound and microbubbles do not have harmful effects on ischemic stroke in MCA occlusion.

Intracranial Perfusion Imaging with Ultrasound in Acute Ischemic Stroke

The assessment of cerebral perfusion is highly relevant for the immediate diagnostic work-up of acute ischemic stroke. MR- and CT-perfusion imaging are routinely used to identify patients who may benefit from recanalizing therapy beyond the standard time window, identifying salvageable tissue at the risk of infarction, e.g. by the MR diffusion-perfusion-based mismatch concept [43]. Other perfusion imaging methods, such as PET-CT and single photon emission computed tomography, are not feasible in acute stroke patients because of logistic limitations. Intracranial perfusion imaging with ultrasound has been shown to be able to identify perfusion deficits of the brain parenchyma in the context of acute ischemic stroke and intracerebral hemorrhage [6, 8, 32, 44, 45]. The advantages of intracranial perfusion imaging with ultrasound are the possibility to perform and repeat the examination at the patient's bedside, allowing for a non-invasive, cheap and quickly applicable assessment of cerebral perfusion at intensive care units or stroke units.

UCA *bolus kinetics* have been analyzed in most of the current perfusion imaging studies of acute ischemic stroke. Different non-linear imaging modalities (harmonic imaging, power modulation, and pulse inversion imaging) with high-MI triggering and different UCAs (Levovist™, Optison™, and SonoVue™) have been used [3, 4, 6, 32, 33, 44, 46–53]. With more sensitive multi-pulse ultrasound technologies, it is possible to analyze brain perfusion not only in the ipsilateral but also in the contralateral hemisphere within one investigation, improving the geometry of the insonation plane and overcoming near-field artifacts [33, 51]. When using this approach, additional artifacts (the calcification of the pineal gland and choroid plexus of the lateral ventricles, causing shadowing artifacts) have to be considered. Different parameters of the (high-MI) bolus kinetics curve acquired from ischemic brain regions in the hyperacute phase of ischemic stroke have been compared with the area of infarction in comparable imaging planes of a follow-up CT. A combination of signal PI reduction compared to the surrounding (healthy) brain tissue and the relative delay in the TTP have been proven to be the most helpful in detecting the area of infarction, with a sensitivity between 75 and 86% as well as a specificity of between 96 and 100% [4, 44].

Several studies have evaluated color-coded parametric images [31, 32]. These images provide information on the time-intensity data of all pixels under evaluation, thus facilitating the visualization and documentation of the perfusion state [31, 33]. Although the supplying artery has been found to be patent by color-coded duplex imaging, in 13–14% of acute ischemic stroke patients, a perfusion deficit in the middle cerebral arterial region could be identified with parametric perfusion imaging [4, 31]. The areas of disturbed perfusion on the parametric images correlate with the area of infarction on the follow-up CT and the severity of stroke symptoms in the early phase as well as the outcome after 4 months [51]. In a pilot study, stroke MRI with diffusion-weighted imaging (DWI) and perfusion-weighted imaging (PWI) maps was used to validate the threshold of PI reduction and TTP delay for the diagnosis of a DWI or PWI lesion [52]. The results of this study showed that an area with isolated PWI delay (without DWI abnormalities = penumbra) could be separated from healthy tissue with the parameters of the wash-in kinetics. For a peak signal with more than one-third of the amplitude of the healthy tissue and a delay of more than 4 s, isolated PWI delay without DWI abnormalities could be suspected.

Spatial resolution for the detection of infarction is a critical point for diagnostic sensitivity. In a study on thalamic infarction, a lesion size of below 2 cm was seldom diagnosed using phase-inversion harmonic imaging [53]. Another critical point in the detection of perfusion deficits in acute ischemic stroke is the time window for detection. A study on ischemic stroke patients in the acute (<12 h) and subacute (>28 h) phases has shown that the detection rate of lesions decreases with time [8]. Reperfusion phenomena may impair the diagnostic impact of later examinations.

Besides contrast bolus kinetics, *destruction kinetics* after the bolus injection of SonoVue™ was evaluated in the early phase of ischemic stroke (<24 h) and compared with perfusion MRI [6]. This pilot study has shown the diagnostic potential of this fast imaging technique to obtain information on regions of reduced perfusion in the early phase of ischemic stroke.

A few studies have examined ultrasound perfusion imaging in patients after hemicraniectomy [46, 48, 54]. In these studies, Doppler-based non-linear imaging technologies with higher receiving frequencies seem to be superior to gray-scale harmonic imaging [33]. In theory, when using high-MI imaging, the direct contrast-enhanced insonation of the brain without the skull (which reduces the actual energy affecting the tissue) could be harmful because of cavitation and capillary rupture [55–57].

Recent reports on the use of low-MI, real-time perfusion imaging in stroke patients have shown that the measurement of real-time *replenishment kinetics* is feasible in patients with sufficient insonation conditions. These analyses have revealed a lower microbubble-refill velocity (β parameter) in ischemic tissue compared to the contralateral normal brain [38]. Moreover, the plateau of acoustic intensity A and the product of A and β as a measure of blood flow also showed significantly lower values in the

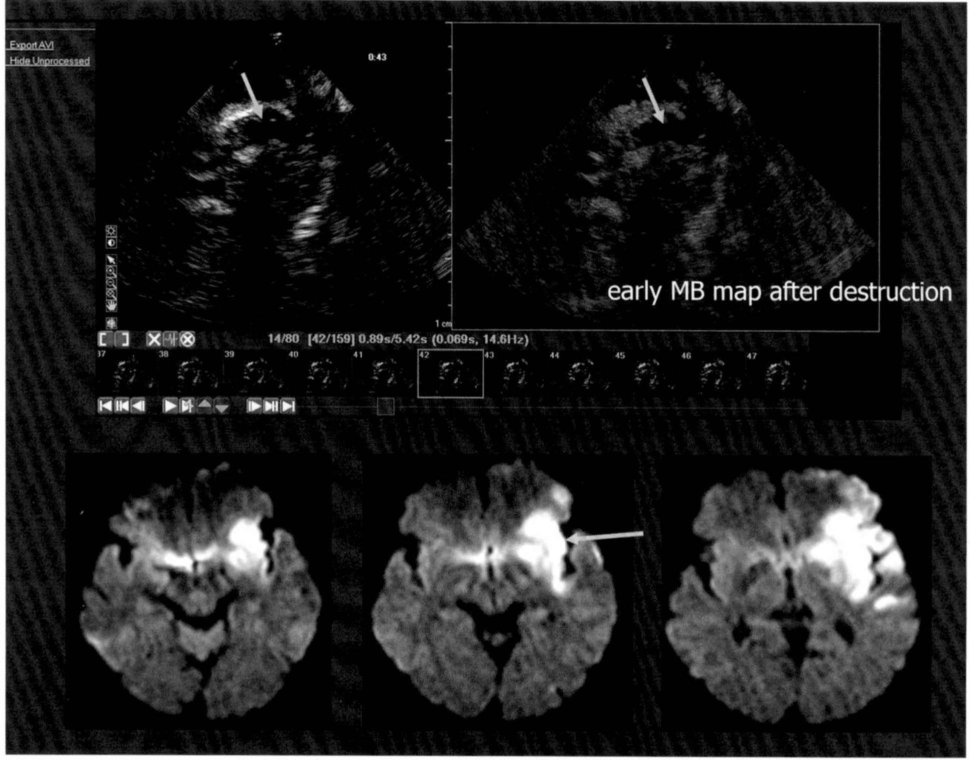

Fig. 6. Microvascular map of left MCA infarction (arrows), which is characterized by absent or diminished contrast agent. The excellent infarction demarcation compares well with the MRI diffusion-weighted imaging (lower images).

ischemic tissue. The findings corresponded with the MRI-derived regional cerebral blood flow maps. A recent study has shown that real-time perfusion imaging can detect hemodynamic impairment in acute MCA occlusion and the subsequent improvement following arterial recanalization. The delay of the TPI was reversible, and the refill parameter β showed a greater slope once the recanalization of the underlying MCA obstruction was demonstrated [58].

Because individual microbubbles can be depicted flowing through small vessels in the brain with low-MI imaging, it is possible to track these bubbles and map perfusion over time using microvascular imaging (MVI). Dynamic MVI maps provide the clear demarcation of MCA infarctions and enable on-line displays of low-velocity tissue microbubble refill following destruction with high-MI imaging [59]. In brain regions showing delayed-contrast bolus arrivals on perfusion-weighted MRI, the ultrasound images show decreased or absent microbubble-refill kinetics (fig. 6). Such findings correlate well with DWI in MRI [59]. Using MVI, the area of maximal perfusion deficit has been compared in patients with brain infarction on follow-up cranial CT with the National Institutes of Health Stroke Scale (NIHSS) score at 24 h after stroke onset.

A significant correlation has been found between the area of maximal perfusion deficit and the NIHSS score at 24 h after symptom onset [60].

Only a few other studies have been undertaken to analyze the correlation between the clinical severity of stroke and the findings of repeated brain perfusion with ultrasound imaging. In a prospective study of 23 patients with acute ischemia in the carotid territory, as analyzed by brain perfusion with harmonic imaging, the area of significant amplitude decrease detected by bolus perfusion harmonic imaging in the early phase of ischemic stroke correlated significantly with the definite area of infarction shown by the follow-up CCT and the outcome of the patient after 4 months [32]. By using pulse-inversion harmonic imaging *(bolus kinetics)* in 27 patients, the sum of the ROIs with 'no perfusion' and 'hypoperfusion' correlated highest with the baseline NIHSS score, and the recruitment of hypoperfused ROIs to the infarction site was highly correlated with the early clinical course [8]. In a recent study of 24 acute stroke patients with a median NIHSS score of 13 and a mean DWI infarct volume of 49.2 ml, clear differences in the perfusion parameters of the bolus kinetics and refill kinetics were shown in the ischemic compared with the non-ischemic brain tissues in patients with the persistent obstruction of the ipsilateral MCA compared with a subgroup of patients with patent MCA. Follow-up examination revealed the normalization of the sonographic parameters along with arterial recanalization [58]. These results indicate that similar to other brain perfusion imaging techniques, the demonstration of changes in microvascular tissue perfusion after spontaneous or after therapeutic reperfusion is feasible with ultrasound brain perfusion imaging. Although perfusion deficits are most accurately detected by ultrasound in the early stages of stroke, when the core of the infarction is able to be differentiated from the viable tissue, follow-up examinations may be useful for monitoring the response to the spontaneous or therapeutic recanalization. These results provide a new opportunity for the bedside monitoring of hemodynamic compromise, e.g. during therapeutic interventions, such as systemic thrombolysis.

References

1 Seidel G, Greis C, Sonne J, Kaps M: Harmonic grey scale imaging of the human brain. J Neuroimaging 1999;9:171–174.
2 Postert T, Muhs A, Meves S, Federlein J, Przuntek H, Buttner T: Transient response harmonic imaging: an ultrasound technique related to brain perfusion. Stroke 1998;29:1901–1907.
3 Meairs S, Daffertshofer M, Neff W, Eschenfelder C, Hennerici M: Pulse-inversion contrast harmonic imaging: ultrasonographic assessment of cerebral perfusion. Lancet 2000;355:550–551.
4 Federlein J, Postert T, Meves S, Weber S, Przuntek H, Buttner T: Ultrasonic evaluation of pathological brain perfusion in acute stroke using second harmonic imaging. J Neurol Neurosurg Psychiatry 2000;69:616–622.
5 Harrer JU, Mayfrank L, Mull M, Klotzsch C: Second harmonic imaging: a new ultrasound technique to assess human brain tumour perfusion. J Neurol Neurosurg Psychiatry 2003;74:333–338.
6 Kern R, Perren F, Schoeneberger K, Gass A, Hennerici M, Meairs S: Ultrasound microbubble destruction imaging in acute middle cerebral artery stroke. Stroke 2004;35:1665–1670.

7 Krogias C, Postert T, Meves S, Wilkening W, Przuntek H, Eyding J: Semiquantitative analysis of ultrasonic cerebral perfusion imaging. Ultrasound Med Biol 2005;31:1007–1012.

8 Eyding J, Krogias C, Schollhammer M, Eyding D, Wilkening W, Meves S, et al: Contrast-enhanced ultrasonic parametric perfusion imaging detects dysfunctional tissue at risk in acute MCA stroke. J Cereb Blood Flow Metab 2006;26:576–582.

9 Wei K, Jayaweera AR, Firoozan S, Linka A, Skyba DM, Kaul S: Quantification of myocardial blood flow with ultrasound-induced destruction of microbubbles administered as a constant venous infusion. Circulation 1998;97:473–483.

10 Schlosser T, Pohl C, Veltmann C, Lohmaier S, Goenechea J, Ehlgen A, et al: Feasibility of the flash-replenishment concept in renal tissue: which parameters affect the assessment of the contrast replenishment? Ultrasound Med Biol 2001;27:937–944.

11 Wei K, Le E, Bin JP, Coggins M, Thorpe J, Kaul S: Quantification of renal blood flow with contrast-enhanced ultrasound. J Am Coll Cardiol 2001;37:1135–1140.

12 Vincent MA, Dawson D, Clark AD, Lindner JR, Rattigan S, Clark MG, et al: Skeletal muscle microvascular recruitment by physiological hyperinsulinemia precedes increases in total blood flow. Diabetes 2002;51:42–48.

13 Postert T, Federlein J, Przuntek H, Buttner T: Insufficient and absent acoustic temporal bone window: potential and limitations of transcranial contrast-enhanced color-coded sonography and contrast-enhanced power-based sonography. Ultrasound Med Biol 1997;23:857–862.

14 Wijnhoud AD, Franckena M, van der Lugt A, Koudstaal PJ, Dippel ED: Inadequate acoustical temporal bone window in patients with a transient ischemic attack or minor stroke: role of skull thickness and bone density. Ultrasound Med Biol 2008;34:923–929.

15 Burns PN. Harmonic imaging with ultrasound contrast agents. Clin Radiol 1996;51(suppl 1):50–55.

16 Della MA, Meyer-Wiethe K, Allemann E, Seidel G: Ultrasound contrast agents for brain perfusion imaging and ischemic stroke therapy. J Neuroimaging 2005;15:217–232.

17 Powers J, Averkiou M, Bruce M: Principles of cerebral ultrasound contrast imaging. Cerebrovasc Dis 2009;27(suppl 2):14–24.

18 Seidel G, Meairs S: Ultrasound contrast agents in ischemic stroke. Cerebrovasc Dis 2009;27(suppl 2):25–39.

19 Pohl C, Tiemann K, Schlosser T, Becher H: Stimulated acoustic emission detected by transcranial color doppler ultrasound: a contrast-specific phenomenon useful for the detection of cerebral tissue perfusion. Stroke 2000;31:1661–1666.

20 Eyding J, Krogias C, Wilkening W, Meves S, Ermert H, Postert T: Parameters of cerebral perfusion in phase-inversion harmonic imaging (PIHI) ultrasound examinations. Ultrasound Med Biol 2003;29:1379–1385.

21 Postert T, Hoppe P, Federlein J, Helbeck S, Ermert H, Przuntek H, et al: Contrast agent specific imaging modes for the ultrasonic assessment of parenchymal cerebral echo contrast enhancement. J Cereb Blood Flow Metab 2000;20:1709–1716.

22 Eyding J, Wilkening W, Reckhardt M, Schmid G, Meves S, Ermert H, et al: Contrast burst depletion imaging (CODIM): a new imaging procedure and analysis method for semiquantitative ultrasonic perfusion imaging. Stroke 2003;34:77–83.

23 Meyer K, Seidel G: Transcranial contrast diminution imaging of the human brain: a pilot study in healthy volunteers. Ultrasound Med Biol 2002;28:1433–1437.

24 Seidel G, Meyer K, Metzler V, Toth D, Vida-Langwasser M, Aach T: Human cerebral perfusion analysis with ultrasound contrast agent constant infusion: a pilot study on healthy volunteers. Ultrasound Med Biol 2002;28:183–189.

25 Eyding J, Wilkening W, Krogias C, Holscher T, Przuntek H, Meves S, et al: Validation of the depletion kinetic in semiquantitative ultrasonographic cerebral perfusion imaging using 2 different techniques of data acquisition. J Ultrasound Med 2004;23:1035–1040.

26 Harrer JU, Klotzsch C: Second harmonic imaging of the human brain: the practicability of coronal insonation planes and alternative perfusion parameters. Stroke 2002;33:1530–1535.

27 Meves SH, Wilkening W, Thies T, Eyding J, Holscher T, Finger M, et al: Comparison between echo contrast agent-specific imaging modes and perfusion-weighted magnetic resonance imaging for the assessment of brain perfusion. Stroke 2002;33:2433–2437.

28 Seidel G, Algermissen C, Christoph A, Katzer T, Kaps M: Visualization of brain perfusion with harmonic gray scale and power doppler technology: an animal pilot study. Stroke 2000;31:1728–1734.

29 Wiesmann M, Seidel G: Ultrasound perfusion imaging of the human brain. Stroke 2000;31:2421–2425.

30 Kern R, Perren F, Kreisel S, Szabo K, Hennerici M, Meairs S: Multiplanar transcranial ultrasound imaging: standards, landmarks and correlation with magnetic resonance imaging. Ultrasound Med Biol 2005;31:311–315.

31 Wiesmann M, Meyer K, Albers T, Seidel G: Parametric perfusion imaging with contrast-enhanced ultrasound in acute ischemic stroke. Stroke 2004;35:508–513.

32 Seidel G, Meyer-Wiethe K, Berdien G, Hollstein D, Toth D, Aach T: Ultrasound perfusion imaging in acute middle cerebral artery infarction predicts outcome. Stroke 2004;35:1107–1111.

33 Eyding J, Nolte-Martin A, Krogias C, Postert T: Changes of contrast-specific ultrasonic cerebral perfusion patterns in the course of stroke; reliability of region-wise and parametric imaging analysis. Ultrasound Med Biol 2007;33:329–334.

34 Holscher T, Wilkening W, Draganski B, Meves SH, Eyding J, Voit H, et al: Transcranial ultrasound brain perfusion assessment with a contrast agent-specific imaging mode: results of a two-center trial. Stroke 2005;36:2283–2285.

35 Sobesky J, Zaro WO, Lehnhardt FG, Hesselmann V, Thiel A, Dohmen C, et al: Which time-to-peak threshold best identifies penumbral flow? A comparison of perfusion-weighted magnetic resonance imaging and positron emission tomography in acute ischemic stroke. Stroke 2004;35:2843–2847.

36 Meyer-Wiethe K, Cangur H, Seidel GU: Comparison of different mathematical models to analyze diminution kinetics of ultrasound contrast enhancement in a flow phantom. Ultrasound Med Biol 2005;31:93–98.

37 Lucidarme O, Kono Y, Corbeil J, Choi SH, Mattrey RF: Validation of ultrasound contrast destruction imaging for flow quantification. Ultrasound Med Biol 2003;29:1697–1704.

38 Kern R, Diels A, Pettenpohl J, Kablau M, Brade J, Hennerici MG, et al: Real-time ultrasound brain perfusion imaging with analysis of microbubble replenishment in acute MCA stroke. J Cereb Blood Flow Metab 2011;31:1716–1724.

39 Rim SJ, Leong-Poi H, Lindner JR, Couture D, Ellegala D, Mason H, et al: Quantification of cerebral perfusion with 'Real-Time' contrast-enhanced ultrasound. Circulation 2001;104:2582–2587.

40 Jungehulsing GJ, Brunecker P, Nolte CH, Fiebach JB, Kunze C, Doepp F, et al: Diagnostic transcranial ultrasound perfusion-imaging at 2.5 MHz does not affect the blood-brain barrier. Ultrasound Med Biol 2008;34:147–150.

41 Stroick M, Alonso A, Fatar M, Griebe M, Kreisel S, Kern R, et al: Effects of simultaneous application of ultrasound and microbubbles on intracerebral hemorrhage in an animal model. Ultrasound Med Biol 2006;32:1377–1382.

42 Fatar M, Stroick M, Griebe M, Alonso A, Kreisel S, Kern R, et al: Effect of combined ultrasound and microbubbles treatment in an experimental model of cerebral ischemia. Ultrasound Med Biol 2008;34: 1414–1420.

43 Schellinger PD, Thomalla G, Fiehler J, Kohrmann M, Molina CA, Neumann-Haefelin T, et al: MRI-based and CT-based thrombolytic therapy in acute stroke within and beyond established time windows: an analysis of 1,210 patients. Stroke 2007;38:2640–2645.

44 Seidel G, Albers T, Meyer K, Wiesmann M: Perfusion harmonic imaging in acute middle cerebral artery infarction. Ultrasound Med Biol 2003;29:1245–1251.

45 Kern R, Kablau M, Sallustio F, Fatar M, Stroick M, Hennerici MG, et al: Improved detection of intracerebral hemorrhage with transcranial ultrasound perfusion imaging. Cerebrovasc Dis 2008;26:277–283.

46 Shiogai T, Takayasu N, Mizuno T, Nakagawa M, Furuhata H: Comparison of transcranial brain tissue perfusion images between ultraharmonic, second harmonic, and power harmonic imaging. Stroke 2004;35:687–693.

47 Postert T, Federlein J, Weber S, Przuntek H, Buttner T: Second harmonic imaging In acute middle cerebral artery infarction. Preliminary results. Stroke 1999;30:1702–1706.

48 Schlachetzki F, Hoelscher T, Dorenbeck U, Greiffenberg B, Marienhagen J, Ullrich O, et al: Sonographic parenchymal and brain perfusion imaging: preliminary results in four patients following decompressive surgery for malignant middle cerebral artery infarct. Ultrasound Med Biol 2001;27:21–31.

49 Stolz E, Allendorfer J, Jauss M, Traupe H, Kaps M: Sonographic harmonic grey scale imaging of brain perfusion: scope of a new method demonstrated in selected cases. Ultraschall Med 2002;23:320–324.

50 Meyer K, Wiesmann M, Albers T, Seidel G: Harmonic imaging in acute stroke: detection of a cerebral perfusion deficit with ultrasound and perfusion MRI. J Neuroimaging 2003;13:166–168.

51 Eyding J, Krogias C, Wilkening W, Postert T: Detection of cerebral perfusion abnormalities in acute stroke using phase inversion harmonic imaging (PIHI): preliminary results. J Neurol Neurosurg Psychiatry 2004;75:926–929.

52 Meyer-Wiethe K, Cangur H, Schindler A, Koch C, Seidel G: Ultrasound perfusion imaging: determination of thresholds for the identification of critically disturbed perfusion in acute ischemic stroke – a pilot study. Ultrasound Med Biol 2007;33:851–856.

53 Nolte CH, Gruss J, Steinbrink J, Jungehulsing GJ, Brunecker P, Hopt AM, et al: Ultrasound perfusion imaging of small stroke involving the thalamus. Ultraschall Med 2009;30:466–470.

54 Bartels E, Bittermann HJ: Transcranial contrast imaging of cerebral perfusion in stroke patients following decompressive craniectomy. Ultraschall Med 2004;25:206–213.

55 Ay T, Havaux X, Van Camp G, Campanelli B, Gisellu G, Pasquet A, et al: Destruction of contrast microbubbles by ultrasound: effects on myocardial function, coronary perfusion pressure, and microvascular integrity. Circulation 2001;104:461–466.

56 Hynynen K, McDannold N, Martin H, Jolesz FA, Vykhodtseva N: The threshold for brain damage in rabbits induced by bursts of ultrasound in the presence of an ultrasound contrast agent (Optison). Ultrasound Med Biol 2003;29:473–481.

57 Hynynen K, McDannold N, Sheikov NA, Jolesz FA, Vykhodtseva N: Local and reversible blood-brain barrier disruption by noninvasive focused ultrasound at frequencies suitable for trans-skull sonications. Neuroimage 2005;24:12–20.

58 Bolognese M, Artemis D, Alonso A, Hennerici MG, Meairs S, Kern R: Real-time ultrasound perfusion imaging in acute stroke: assessment of cerebral perfusion deficits related to arterial recanalization. Ultrasound Med Biol 2013;39:745–752.

59 Pettenpohl J, Diels A, Kablau M, Kern R, Sick C, Hennerici M, et al: Dynamic microvascular perfusion maps for assessement of brain infarction. Cerebrovasc Dis 2007;23:16.

60 Seidel G, Roessler F, Al-Khaled M: Microvascular imaging in acute ischemic stroke. J Neuroimaging 2013;23:166–169.

Prof. Stephen Meairs, MD, PhD
Department of Neurology
Universitätsmedizin Mannheim, University of Heidelberg
Theodor-Kutzer-Ufer 1–3, DE–68167 Mannheim (Germany)
E-Mail meairs@neuro.ma.uni-heidelberg.de

Alonso A, Hennerici MG, Meairs S (eds): Translational Neurosonology.
Front Neurol Neurosci. Basel, Karger, 2015, vol 36, pp 71–82 (DOI: 10.1159/000366238)

Parenchymal Imaging in Movement Disorders

Rita de Cássia Leite Fernandes[a] · Daniela Berg[b]

[a]Department of Neurology, University Hospital Clementino Fraga Filho, Federal University of Rio de Janeiro,
10º andar – Cidade Universitária, Rio de Janeiro, Brazil; [b]Department of Neurodegeneration at the UKT, Hertie
Institut of Clinical Brain Research and German Center for Neurodegenerative Diseases, Tübingen, Germany

Abstract

The use of B-mode sonography in neurological diagnosis was once considered of limited importance
due to the barrier of the skull. However, modern ultrasound systems allow visualization of the brain
parenchyma with a high degree of accuracy. Transcranial sonography (TCS) can offer unique information on brain tissue pathology, as it uses different physical principles for imaging acquisition than
do other neuroimaging techniques. The method is harmless, is quick to perform at low cost and demands no sedation. The main limitations of this technique are dependence on the quality of the
individual bone window and on proper operator training. A huge body of research has shown that
patients with Parkinson's disease (PD) display an enlarged hyperechogenic substantia nigra by TCS
with a positive predictive value of 92.9%. Healthy individuals (8–15%) may show the same marker,
in some cases correlating with decreased striatal dopamine uptake, motor slowing and prodromal
markers of PD, indicating that this ultrasound sign may constitute a risk marker for PD. Other movement disorder diagnoses, although less extensively studied for TCS, may benefit from using this
method as a supplementary diagnostic tool. This review provides a summary of the typical TCS findings and their value in the differential diagnosis of some movement disorders.

© 2015 S. Karger AG, Basel

Introduction

For more than five decades, the ultrasound technique has progressed towards being
a well-established diagnostic method in general medicine. However, in the fields of
neurology and neurosurgery, ultrasound has only relatively recently been introduced into clinical practice. This delay is likely due to the hindering of the passage
of acoustic waves due to the osseous barrier of the skull bones. It was only in 1982
that Aaslid et al. [1] reported capturing Doppler signals from the middle and ante-

rior cerebral arteries, as perceived via scanning through the temporal bone window with a 2-MHz pulsed Doppler. This discovery ushered in the era of non-invasive investigation of intracranial vascular disease. Studying the brain parenchyma using two-dimensional sonography had to wait until the last decade of the 20th century. In 1995, German investigators, led by Georg Becker [2], published the first report of an alteration at the mesencephalic substantia nigra (SN), which was depicted by B-mode sonography, in patients with Parkinson's disease (PD). This group stated that the region at the anatomical site of the SN was much more echogenic in PD patients compared to individuals without PD and that this finding could be a useful neuroimaging marker for the disease. This astonishing finding was perceived with skepticism, as other structural neuroimaging methods, such as CT or MRI, were not capable of visualizing alterations typical of PD. However, scientific curiosity, the easy applicability of the method at low cost, the lack of side effects and the lack of discomfort during the investigation overcame this reluctance and piqued the interest of the scientific community. In the last 19 years, transcranial sonography (TCS) has thus been utilized in research, as well as in clinical routine in some centers, in the assessment of characteristic abnormalities of the substantia nigra, midbrain raphe, basal ganglia, and cerebral ventricles in various movement disorders [3].

TCS depicts echogenic, deep brain structures with high resolution [4] and has many important advantages. First, it is based on different physical principles than are other imaging techniques. Therefore, TCS can offer unique and complementary information on brain tissue pathology. Economically speaking, ultrasound equipment is much lower in cost than other imaging alternatives. The machines are generally widely available in health facilities where the same transducers are already used to perform transcranial Doppler. Moreover, bedside exams are a possibility, given that several types of ultrasound devices are relatively portable. Importantly, ultrasound only requires a short examination time and can be used in anxious patients. Because the investigator is able to compensate for the patient's involuntary movements, there is also no need for sedation, and its inherent risks are low. Finally, the harmlessness of TCS allows for unlimited scans without the danger of radiation. Thus, ultrasound can be regarded as a convenient imaging technique that provides helpful supplementary information of the brain in healthy and diseased states. As with any imaging method, there are some limitations to ultrasound. The technique depends on the quality of the individual acoustic bone windows, and it provides poor access to brain regions near the insonating probe, basal skull bones and high frontoparietal regions. Ultrasound is also an operator-dependent technique, requiring proper training and experience for good data acquisition and interpretation [3].

For each of the following movement disorders, a comprehensive summary of the typical findings that have been acquired with TCS are described, and their values in diagnosis and differential diagnosis are provided.

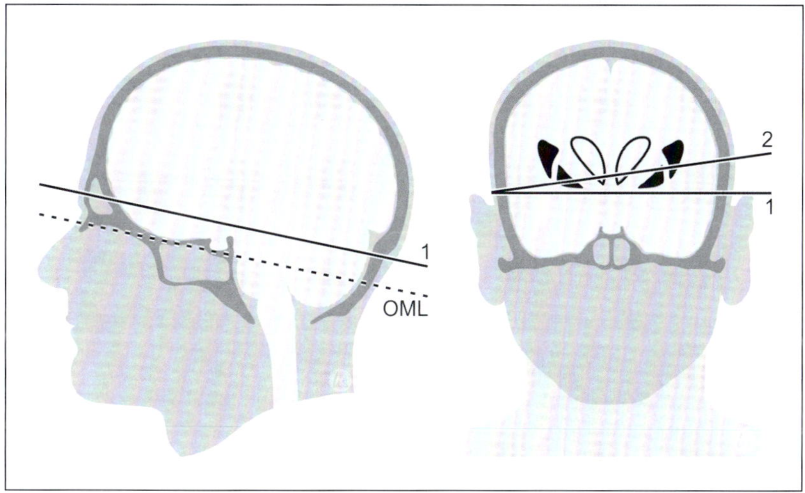

Fig. 1. Standardized planes of transcranial sonography. OML = Orbitomeatal line; Line 1 = mesence-phalic plane; Line 2 = basal ganglia plane.

Methods

The exam is performed through the acoustic bone window in front of the ear (fig. 1). At this site, the temporal bone is thinner, allowing sound waves of low frequency to penetrate and reach the deep structures of the brain. In about 80–90% of the Caucasian population, the optimal quality of the bone window allows good visualization of all structures of interest when all age groups are considered. A higher prevalence of poor windows has been reported in elderly patients, women, and individuals of Asian descent [3, 5].

An optimized ultrasound system equipped with a low frequency (1–3 MHz), phased-array transducer should be used. A penetration depth of 14–16 cm allows for visualization of the contralateral skull bone when the focus is set in the middle of the image. The dynamic range should be set at 45–55 dB, with medium or high-contour amplification. Image brightness and time-gain compensation are individually adapted during each scan as needed. Tissue harmonic imaging allows for a more distinct depiction of tissue interfaces and may be used to improve resolution, but its dependency on the bone window prevents its more generalized use. Moreover, the size of structures seems exaggerated using tissue harmonic imaging [6].

The patient is placed in the supine position, and the investigator approaches both temporal windows from behind the head. The two scanning planes that are routinely used for the evaluation of relevant brain structures in movement disorders are the mesencephalic plane and the basal ganglia plane. Eventually, a cerebellar plane may also be used.

Mesencephalic Brainstem Plane
The examination starts in the axial scanning plane parallel to the so-called 'orbitomeatal line' to depict the key structures within this horizontal plane (fig. 2). At the center of the image, one finds the black (hypoechoic), butterfly-shaped mesencephalon contrasting with the surrounding white (hyperechoic) basal cisterns.

By convention, the dorsal structures are displayed to the right, and the structures ipsilateral to the insonating probe are visualized at the superior part of the image. The nigral area is found in each cerebral peduncle and runs on an oblique, medio-lateral axis. Normally, the SN is depicted as

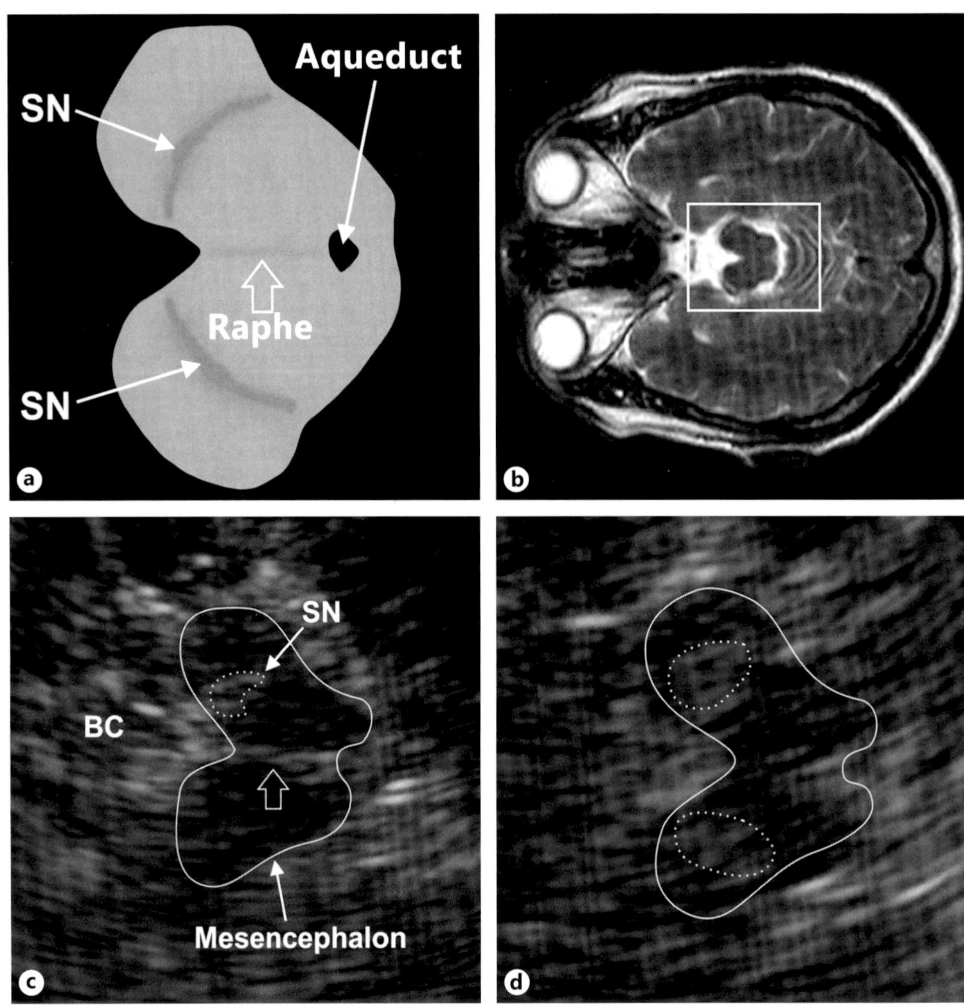

Fig. 2. Mesencephalic images by magnetic resonance imaging and transcranial sonography (TCS). **a** Schematic illustration of the midbrain structures. SN = Substantia nigra. **b** MRI corresponding to the image in **c** and **d**. The square denotes the area to be evaluated using sonography. **c** Normal TCS (axial scanning plane) at the orbitomeatal line showing the hypoechoic mesencephalon surrounded by hyperechoic basal cisterns (BC). The brainstem is divided by the hyperechogenic raphe line (open arrow). A normal SN at the ipsilateral peduncle is encircled. **d** TCS showing enlarged bilateral SN areas of echogenicity (= hyperechogenicity) at the anatomical site of the SN in a Parkinson's disease patient.

a thin, echogenic, sometimes rather patchy line. The echogenicity of the SN used to be graded semi-quantitatively as isoechogenic, mildly echogenic, and hyperechogenic with regard to the surrounding mesencephalon. In contrast to this subjective evaluation, the planimetrically measured area of nigral echogenicity has been used more often because it allows for better comparison across observers and studies, thus enhancing the reproducibility of the method [5, 6]. After freezing and zooming, the SN echogenic area is manually encircled on the ipsilateral peduncle for the planimetrically area measurement. SN areas <0.20 cm^2 are defined as normal because they represent 75% of the

Fernandes · Berg

areas found in the normal population. Sizes between 0.20 and 0.25 cm^2 are classified as moderately enlarged, and sizes $\geq$0.25 cm^2, representing the upper 10th percentile of the normal population, are denoted as markedly enlarged [7]. Because the lateral resolution depends on the width of the ultrasonic beam, the distribution of normal SN area values should be determined for specific ultrasound equipment, populations and laboratories [4, 6].

A recent paper addressed the issue of validity and argued that the method has an excellent intrarater and interrater reproducibility when the measurements are obtained by experienced investigators [5].

The other important structure to be rated at this plane is the hyperechogenic line that crosses the mesencephalon in an anterior-posterior direction and represents the nuclei and fiber tracts of the raphe system. The raphe line is rated semi-quantitatively as normal (continuous) or abnormal (non-continuous or absent) [6].

Basal Ganglia Plane
The basal ganglia plane is reached by tilting the ultrasound probe slightly (10–20°) upward starting from the midbrain plane (fig. 3). At this level, the intensively echogenic pineal gland, identified at the dorsal part of the image, serves as a landmark. The midline third ventricle is delineated by the two hyperechoic, parallel lines of its walls. The width of the third ventricle should be measured in frozen and magnified images at the largest diameter by placing the calipers at the inner surfaces of the ependyma. Ventral to the third ventricle, the comma-shaped frontal horn of the lateral ventricle contralateral to the insonating probe can be measured perpendicularly between the medial (septum pellucid) and distal walls. For individuals younger than 60 years, the maximum measurement values are 7 mm for the third ventricle and 17 mm for the anterior horns. For those older than 60 years, measurements should not exceed 10 and 20 mm, respectively [3, 6].

The thalamus is in general even less echogenic than the basal ganglia, particularly the lentiform nuclei (LN) and caudate nuclei (CN), which are normally isoechogenic to the surrounding brain tissue, with the CN being slightly more echogenic than the LN. These structures, which are adjacent to the midline ventricle, are also evaluated contralateral to the insonating probe, as resolution close to the probe is limited due to the wavelength. Any hyperechogenic focus found at this anatomical site should be measured and registered because it may represent a pathological condition [6].

Transcranial Sonography in the Diagnosis of Movement Disorders

Parkinson's Disease and Parkinsonian Syndromes
Until now, the gold standard for PD diagnosis has been the recognition of PD-specific pathology in the post-mortem neuropathological exam. Despite the absence of a biological marker, the clinical diagnosis of idiopathic PD made by movement disorder specialists is very accurate in patients with long-standing, typical features such as asymmetric resting tremor, bradykinesia, rigidity, and good therapeutic response to levodopa [8]. However, in the early stages, it may be very difficult to differentiate PD from the atypical Parkinsonisms, including multiple system atrophy (MSA), progressive supranuclear palsy (PSP), corticobasal degeneration, and diffuse Lewy body disease. All of these diseases are characterized by a Parkinsonian syndrome with additional features such as autonomic symptoms, supranuclear gaze palsy, lack of levodopa responsiveness, and rapid progression. Another subset of diseases in the differential

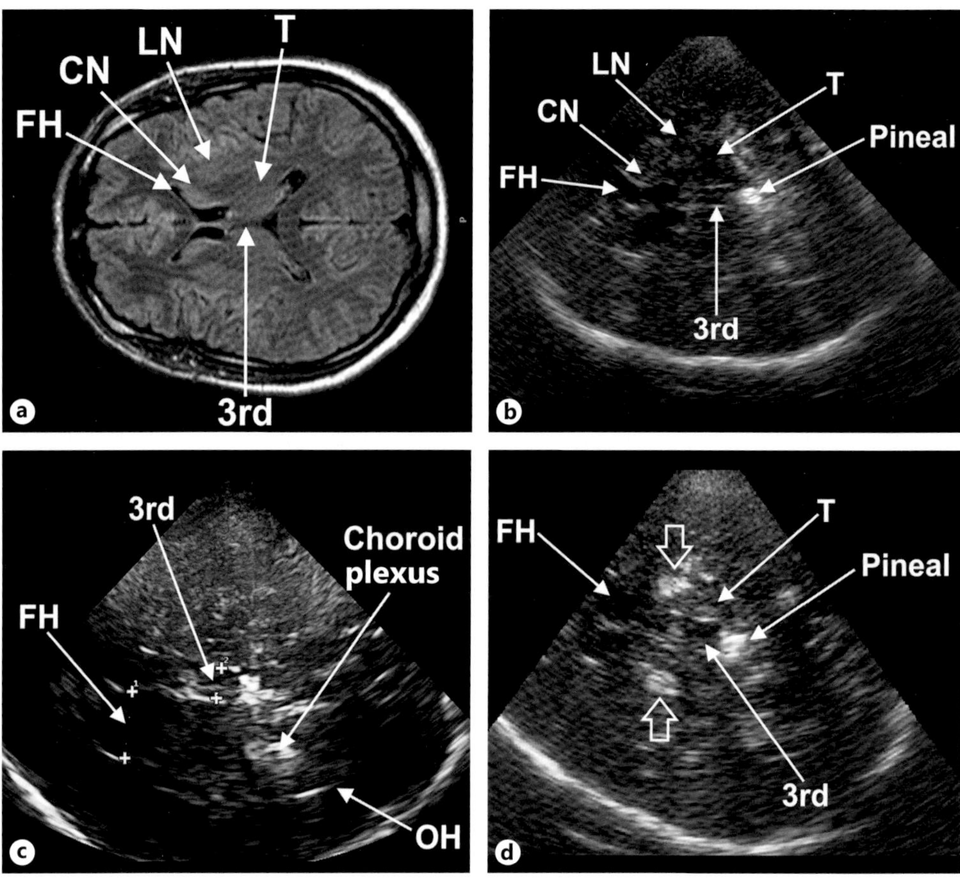

Fig. 3. Basal ganglia plane using magnetic resonance imaging and transcranial sonography (TCS). **a** Magnetic resonance imaging depiction of the corresponding structures. **b** Normal basal ganglia plane by TCS. **c** TCS image at the basal ganglia plane depicting ventricular enlargement (3rd ventricle = 11.3 mm; frontal horn of lateral ventricle = 25.0 mm). The occipital horn of the contralateral lateral ventricle, with the choroid plexus inside, is also depicted. **d** TCS image showing bilateral areas of hyperechogenicity at the lentiform nucleus (opened arrows). CN = Caudate nucleus; FH = frontal horn of the lateral ventricle; LN = lentiform nucleus; OH = occipital horn of the lateral ventricle; T = thalamus; 3rd = third ventricle.

diagnosis of PD are secondary Parkinsonisms, including vascular and drug-induced Parkinsonism, hydrocephalus, depression, and disorders of heavy metal accumulation, such as Wilson's disease (WD). An important differential diagnosis for tremor-dominant PD is essential tremor (ET). An early, correct diagnosis is of cardinal importance, as prognosis and management differ considerably among these various conditions. Thus, a reliable imaging marker is of great importance [3, 7].

TCS enables visualization of a neuroimaging marker of PD with high sensitivity. It has been demonstrated in numerous papers published worldwide that patients with idiopathic PD display an enlarged echogenic area at the anatomical site of the SN that is 0.20 cm^2 or larger (SN+) in 68–99% of PD cases [9], with a positive predictive value of 92.9% in cases of early Parkinsonism (fig. 2d) [10]. The differences in prevalence found across studies can be ascribed to methodological issues such as differing cut-off values for abnormal SN area, the equipment used, and the ethnic background of the studied population [6, 9].

The extension of the SN echogenic area was found to be larger contralateral to the side with more severe symptoms and stable with disease progression [11]. However, some authors have found a moderate positive correlation between the nigral area and the duration of the disease [12, 13], while others could not support this finding [14]. Thus, SN+ seems to be a sensible marker for the diagnosis of idiopathic PD but not for monitoring disease progression, although there is no consensus on this last issue.

It has been reported that 8–15% of healthy people undergoing TCS are SN+ [11], which impacts the diagnostic accuracy and specificity of the method [5]. Some of these individuals show decreased striatal ^{18}F-Dopa uptake, as measured by PET [15]. Moreover, SN+ has been found to be more prevalent in older age groups, likely relating to motor slowing in the elderly [3]. Interestingly, the frequency of this SN feature in the healthy population fits well with the 17% prevalence of incidental nigral Lewy Bodies that has been found in asymptomatic persons aged older than 80 years [16]. All of these data support the theory that SN hyperechogenicity could be also a marker for subclinical nigrostriatal alterations and increased susceptibility to PD [17]. A recent prospective study reported a substantially higher relative risk for incidental PD among at-baseline, PD-free individuals with SN+ when compared to participants with normoechogenic SN [18]. Thus, the echofeature could serve as a premotor marker for PD.

A hyperechogenic focus in the LN can be found in 79% of atypical Parkinsonian cases (fig. 3d) but considerably less often in PD (23%) or healthy controls (6%) [9]. Moreover, SN+ is found less frequently in MSA and PSP. Therefore, SN+ associated with a normal echogenicity of the LN is strongly suggestive for idiopathic PD. Conversely, a normal SN echogenic area and a hyperechogenic signal of the LN raises a red flag for the possibility of MSA or PSP. Additionally, third ventricle dilation may favor the diagnosis of PSP [3], but large ventricles and a normal SN area also raise the possibility of hydrocephalus (fig. 3c) [3, 11]. Some diagnostic uncertainty may arise from two rare disorders, DLB and corticobasal degeneration, which show Lewy body pathology in addition to SN+ in an impressive number of cases [6].

The Parkinsonian features developed by some patients after the use of anti-dopaminergic drugs (e.g., neuroleptics, calcium channel blockers) are usually not accompanied by abnormalities on TCS. However, the presence of SN+ in a subset of these patients raises the question as to whether they are candidates for the future development of PD [11].

The prevalence of SN+ among depressive patients follows a gradient, as they exhibit this feature more frequently than healthy individuals but less frequently than PD patients [11]. Another echofeature that may help to further differentiate PD from depression is the abnormal appearance of the midbrain raphe [6]. It has been found that the raphe line is absent or interrupted in 50–70% of depressed individuals; however, an interrupted or missing raphe line is also frequently found in PD patients with depression (40–60%). It seems that only a combination of TCS findings (e.g., normal SN echogenicity plus abnormal midline raphe) would be able to correctly differentiate these two conditions in the clinical setting. As depression constitutes a known premotor marker of PD, the presence of SN+ may disclose those depressive individuals as at-risk for later development of PD [3].

Essential Tremor

The occurrence of the echomarker SN+ among ET patients is more frequent than in healthy individuals but less frequent than in PD patients [6]. A systematic review on the subject found that TCS differentiated PD from ET with a sensitivity of 75–86% [9]. A study using [123I]-FP-CIT single photon emission computed tomography as the imaging gold standard has confirmed that TCS allows reliable differentiation between PD and ET [19].

As the risk for subsequent development of PD is about three- to four-times higher in ET patients, one could speculate that ET patients with SN+ may constitute a higher-risk group for PD [11].

Dystonia

Idiopathic dystonia, medication-induced dystonia, and psychogenic disorders mimicking dystonia may have normal CT and MRI findings and constitute a major differential diagnostic challenge to the neurologist. One report found hyperechogenic lesions in the LN in more than 75% of idiopathic dystonia patients (fig. 3d) [20]. Based on post-mortem studies, it was proposed that an elevated regional copper content, which was found using TCS, could constitute the pathophysiological basis for dystonia [21]. A more recent study, however, found LN hyperechogenicity in more than 50% of patients affected by cervical dystonia but also in half of their controls [22]. The authors considered this an unspecific signal due to its high prevalence in the controls.

Restless Leg Syndrome

Restless leg syndrome (RLS) is a common neurologic condition that is characterized by an urge to move the legs that occurs at rest and is relieved by movement. A study described decreased SN echogenicity (SN-) in patients with RLS with good sensitivity (82%), specificity (83%), and positive predictive value (94%) [23]. Midline raphe hypoechogenicity was shown to be more prevalent in RLS patients than in controls and was correlated with depression and periodic limb movements. The combination of these features indicated RLS with a positive predictive value of 97% [11].

The area of SN echogenicity was shown to also be smaller in Friedreich's ataxia (FA) patients and significantly associated with the occurrence of RLS symptomatology. A prevalence of SN- was found to be significantly higher in FA patients (44%) than in controls (11.8%) [24]. Nigral iron deficiency in these FA patients was suggested as a plausible explanation for their SN hypoechogenicity [11].

Wilson's Disease

Walter and colleagues [25] investigated 21 patients with neurologically symptomatic (n = 18) or asymptomatic WD. LN hyperechogenicity was found in all neurologically symptomatic patients as well as in two of three asymptomatic individuals. Disease severity correlated with the sizes of the LN and thalamus hyperechogenic focus as well as with the widths of the third and lateral ventricles. A more recent work evaluated 54 patients with WD in which TCS revealed significantly higher prevalence of SN and LN hyperechogenicity when compared to controls [26]. Disease severity was correlated with the SN echogenic area and with the width of the third ventricle.

Both studies demonstrate the ability of TCS to detect the accumulation of copper and perhaps other trace metals in the basal ganglia of WD patients, including pre-symptomatic subjects in whom CT and MRI failed to show abnormalities.

Huntington's Disease

Postert et al. demonstrated hyperechogenic lesions in the basal ganglia in more than a third of 45 patients with HD, a characteristic that was only found in 12.8% of controls [27]. SN+ correlated positively with the number of CAG repetitions, and six patients (13.3%) showed marked CN hyperechogenicity, a feature that is usually not described in healthy people. The work of Krogias et al. also reported a significantly higher percentage of SN+ (41%) and CN hyperechogenicity (20.6%) in 39 patients with HD when compared to controls (17.5 and 5%, respectively) [28]. In 71.4% of the patients with depressive symptoms, the brainstem raphe was pathological. The width of the third ventricle was markedly enlarged in HD patients, which correlated well with the CT findings, correlated inversely with the cognitive score, and could be caused by thalamic atrophy.

These two studies on TCS in HD show comparable results and demonstrate that TCS may provide reliable information about brain morphology, even in agitated HD patients who do not tolerate other imaging techniques.

Causes of Abnormal Echogenicity of Regions of the Brain Parenchyma

To date, the reason for the abnormal echo pattern of brain structures depicted by TCS is not entirely clear. In general, increased echogenicity mirrors increased impedance at tissue interfaces. In PD, this pattern can be the result of microglia proliferation and increased heavy metal tissue content, especially iron [7]. Previous postmortem and neurochemical studies have revealed a close correlation between SN echogenicity and tissue iron content [17]. In addition, experiments in rats have demonstrated that more intense tissue echogenicity is induced by injecting increasing amounts of iron into the SN [3, 6].

Further support for this iron hypothesis comes from the opposed changes in nigral echogenicity that is observed in PD and RLS. While hyperechogenicity is a typical feature of PD due to a suspected increase in the nigral iron content, hypoechogenicity has primarily been demonstrated in RLS, a condition that is associated with low iron concentrations in brainstem structures [11].

Deposits of copper have also been implicated in changes in brain parenchyma echogenicity, as in WD [25] and dystonia [21]. Striopallidodentate calcinosis with extensively hyperechogenic signals at the basal ganglia, as depicted by TCS, has been described, suggesting that calcium deposits may also contribute to changes in the normal echogenic patterns of brain structures [3].

New Directions

Despite its proven clinical relevance, TCS is still restricted to movement disorder clinics and is seldom performed by neuroradiologists [4]. One reason for this reluctance is the difficulty in subjectively identifying the changes in tissue echogenicity without considerable experience in the field. To overcome this limitation, new approaches for the automatic quantification of SN echogenicity are highly desirable [29].

Another important future application of TCS is the visualization of deep brain stimulation electrodes. Walter et al. [30] found TCS to be a reliable method for the detection of lead dislocation requiring reinsertion. A favorable 12-month clinical outcome was associated with optimal lead location, as defined by a TCS scan. Given the disadvantages inherent to other neuroimaging methods in these cases (e.g., radiation exposure, artifacts generated by metal tips, heating of the electrodes), TCS may represent a quick, reliable, and safe alternative.

Conclusions

As suggested by the above-mentioned body of research, we anticipate that B-mode sonography of the brain parenchyma will become a valuable method in everyday neurological practice for the differential diagnosis of Parkinsonian syndromes. However, further studies need to show the relevance of this method to the premotor diagnosis of PD and deep brain stimulation electrode location. In addition to possessing the distinct advantages of portability, low cost, no sedation requirement, and lack of biological side effects, TCS provides the physician with valuable additional information and clues in the investigation of movement disorders. General disadvantages of TCS are its dependency on the temporal window and skill of the investigator, but new methodologies aimed at a more objective assessment of TCS images may overcome these limitations in the near future.

References

1 Aaslid R, Markwalder TM, Nornes H: Noninvasive transcranial Doppler ultrasound recording of flow velocity in basal cerebral arteries. J Neurosurg 1982; 57:769–774.

2 Becker G, Seufert J, Bogdahn U, et al: Degeneration of substantia nigra in chronic Parkinson's disease visualized by transcranial color-coded real-time sonography. Neurology 1995;45:182–184.

3 Berg D, Steinberger JD, Olanow WC, et al: Milestones in magnetic resonance imaging and Transcranial sonography of movement disorders. Mov Disord 2011;26:979–992.

4 Walter U, Kanowski M, Kaufmann J, et al: Contemporary ultrasound systems allow high-resolution transcranial imaging of small echogenic deep intracranial structures similarly as MRI: a phantom study. Neuroimage 2008;40:551–558.

5 van de Loo S, Walter U, Behnke S, et al: Reproducibility and diagnostic accuracy of substantia nigra sonography for the diagnosis of Parkinson's disease. J Neurol Neurosurg Psychiatry 2010;81:1087–1092.

6 Walter U, Behnke S, Eyding J, et al: Transcranial brain parenchyma sonography in movement disorders: state of the art. Ultrasound Med Biol 2007;33: 15–25.

7 Berg D, Siefker C, Becker G: Echogenicity of the substantia nigra in Parkinson's disease and its relation to clinical findings. J Neurol 2001;248:684–689.

8 Hughes AJ, Daniel SE, Ben-Shlomo Y, et al: The accuracy of diagnosis of parkinsonian syndromes in a specialist movement disorder service. Brain 2002; 125:861–870.

9 Vlaar AMM, Bouwmans A, Mess WH, et al: Transcranial duplex in the differential diagnosis of parkinsonian syndromes: a systematic review. J Neurology 2009;256:530–538.

10 Gaenslen A, Unmuth B, Godau J, et al: The specificity and sensitivity of transcranial ultrasound in the differential diagnosis of Parkinson's disease: a prospective blinded study. Lancet Neurol 2008;7:417–424.

11 Godau J, Berg D: Role of transcranial ultrasound in the diagnosis of movement disorders. Neuroimaging Clin N Am 2010;20:87–101.

12 Tsai CF, Wu RM, Huang YW, et al: Transcranial color-coded sonography helps differentiation between idiopathic Parkinson's disease and vascular parkinsonism. J Neurol 2007;254:501–507.

13 Weise D, Lorenz R, Schliesser M, et al: Substantia nigra echogenicity: a structural correlate of functional impairment of the dopaminergic striatal projection in Parkinson's disease. Mov Disord 2009;24: 1669–1675.

14 Behnke S, Runkel A, Kassar HA-S, et al: Long-term course of substantia nigra hyperechogenicity in Parkinson's disease. Mov Disord 2013;28:455–459.

15 Behnke S, Schroeder U, Dillmann U, et al: Hyperechogenicity of the substantia nigra in healthy controls is related to MRI changes and to neuronal loss as determined by F-Dopa PET. Neuroimage 2009;47: 1237–1243.

16 Buchman AS, Shulman JM, Sukriti N, et al: Nigral pathology and parkinsonian signs in elders without Parkinson disease. Ann Neurol 2012;71:258–266.

17 Berg D, Roggendorf W, Schröder U, et al: Echogenicity of the substantia nigra: association with increased iron content and marker for susceptibility to nigrostriatal injury. Arch Neurol 2002;59:999–1005.

18 Berg D, Behnke S, Seppi K, et al: Enlarged hyperechogenic substantia nigra as a risk marker for Parkinson's disease. Mov Disord 2013;28:216–219.

19 Doepp F, Plotkin M, Siegel L, et al: Brain parenchyma sonography and 123I-FP-CIT SPECT in Parkinson's disease and essential tremor. Mov Disord 2008; 23:405–410.

20 Naumann M, Becker G, Toyka KV, et al: Lenticular nucleus lesion in idiopathic dystonia detected by transcranial sonography. Neurology 1996;47:1284–1290.

21 Becker G, Berg D, Francis M, et al: Evidence for disturbances of copper metabolism in dystonia: from the image towards a new concept. Neurology 2001; 57:2290–2294.

22 Hagenah J, König IR, Kötter C, et al: Basal ganglia hyperechogenicity does not distinguish between patients with primary dystonia and healthy individuals. J Neurol 2011;258:590–595.

23 Godau J, Wevers AK, Gaenslen A, et al: Sonographic abnormalities of brainstem structures in restless legs syndrome. Sleep Med 2008;9:782–789.

24 Stockner H, Sojer M, Hering S, et al: Substantia nigra hypoechogenicity in Friedreich ataxia. Mov Disord 2012;27:332–333.

25 Walter U, Krolikowski K, Tarnacka B, et al: Sonographic detection of basal ganglia lesions in asymptomatic and symptomatic Wilson disease. Neurology 2005;64:1726–1732.

26 Svetel M, Mijajlović M, Tomić A, et al: Transcranial sonography in Wilson's disease. Parkinsonism Relat Disord 2012;18:234–238.

27 Postert T, Lack B, Kuhn W, et al: Basal ganglia alterations and brain atrophy in Huntington's disease depicted by transcranial real time sonography. J Neurol Neurosurg Psychiatry 1999;67:457–462.

28 Krogias C, Strassburger K, Eyding J, et al: Depression in patients with Huntington disease correlates with alterations of the brain stem raphe depicted by transcranial sonography. J Psychiatry Neurosci 2011;36:187–194.

29 Fernandes RCL, Rosso ALZ, Vincent MB, et al: Transcranial sonography of substantia nigra: computer-evaluated echogenicity. Mov Disord 2012;27(suppl 1):S235.

30 Walter U, Kirsch M, Wittstock M, et al: Transcranial sonographic localization of deep brain stimulation electrodes is safe, reliable and predicts clinical outcome. Ultrasound Med Biol 2011;37:1382–1391.

Dr. Rita de Cássia Leite Fernandes
Serviço de Neurologia, Hospital Universitário Clementino Fraga Filho
Rua Prof° Rodolpho Paulo Rocco, 255, sala 10E36, Cidade Universitária
Rio de Janeiro 21941-913 (Brazil)
E Mail ritafernandes@ufrj.br

Fernandes · Berg

Alonso A, Hennerici MG, Meairs S (eds): Translational Neurosonology.
Front Neurol Neurosci. Basel, Karger, 2015, vol 36, pp 83–93 (DOI: 10.1159/000366239)

Sonothrombolysis

Stephen Meairs

Department of Neurology, Universitätsmedizin Mannheim, University of Heidelberg, Mannheim, Germany

Abstract

Ultrasound (US) applied as an adjunct to thrombolytic therapy improves the recanalization of occluded vessels, and microbubbles can amplify this effect. New data suggests that the combination of US and microbubbles without tissue plasminogen activator may achieve recanalization with a lower risk of hemorrhage. Further possibilities include specific targeting of thrombus with immunobubbles as well as local drug delivery with US-sensitive liposomes. Clinical studies support the use of US for ischemic stroke therapy, and the first trials of enhancing sonothrombolysis with microbubbles have been encouraging. One emerging clinical application is sonothrombolysis of intracranial hemorrhages for clot evacuation. Microcirculation, irrespective of recanalization, may also be improved by US and microbubbles, and this effect may open new opportunities for the application of sonothrombolysis in acute ischemic stroke. Understanding the mechanisms of therapeutic action and relating this knowledge to issues of efficacy and safety are important objectives of ongoing research. This review will discuss the translational capacities of in vitro studies and preclinical research and will assess the first clinical studies of this promising therapeutic strategy.

© 2015 S. Karger AG, Basel

Experimental Evidence for Clot Lysis with Ultrasound

Historical Perspective

In 1974, Sobbe et al. [1] applied 26.5-kHz ultrasound (US) to recanalize thrombosed iliofemoral arteries in dogs. In the following years, several studies showed that catheter-based or transcutaneous US could enhance the effect of fibrinolytic agents in recanalizing thrombosed arteries [2–8]. These pioneering efforts paved the way for the first clinical studies evaluating the adjunct effect of US in treating patients with ischemic stroke.

Mechanisms of Ultrasound Thrombolysis
Despite numerous studies documenting a thrombolytic effect of US, the mechanisms of this effect remain poorly understood. Inertial cavitation (i.e. the formation and violent collapse of gas-filled bubbles in a fluid exposed to US) gives rise to transient microjets that mechanically disintegrate the thrombus [9]. Stable cavitation (i.e. sustainable, nonlinear, periodic contraction or expansion of a gas body or bubble) may be more effective in clot lysis than inertial cavitation [10]. US also facilitates the penetration of fibrinolytic drugs into the thrombus and the binding to fibrin [11] because US promotes the motion of fluids around the clot surface through a process called microstreaming. Moreover, pressure waves may increase the permeation of tissue plasminogen activator (t-PA) into the interior of the fibrin network [12]. Heating is uniformly present in tissue exposed to US but has been deemed too mild to explain the thrombolytic effects.

Microbubble-Enhanced Thrombolysis with Tissue Plasminogen Activator
Significant amplification of lysis occurs with the addition of microbubbles to the thrombolytic drug and US combination [13–15]. Microbubbles, which are composed of lipid, albumin, or galactose shells and range in size from 0.5–5 µm, lower the threshold for thrombolysis by providing a preexisting bubble that can easily be made to cavitate by US. Stable cavitation can produce microstreaming in the area and dramatically enlarge the bubble momentarily, which will cause localized mechanical stress on the adjacent clot. The surface of the clot will erode, and penetration and numerous microscopic holes inside the clot have been demonstrated [9]. Microstreaming also leads to a dramatic increase in the delivery of a thrombolytic drug to the clot [16]. More energy delivered to the microbubble can lead to inertial cavitation, which ends with violent disruption of the bubble and can produce microjets that are also effective in eroding the clot [17]. Pressure waves interact with the bubbles, causing expansion and contraction, which can lead to 'pumping' of energy from the traveling wave and 'focusing' and re-emitting the wave locally, sometimes at other, perhaps better frequencies.

Clot Lysis with Ultrasound and Microbubbles
A number of studies have reported successful thrombolysis with microbubbles and US alone, i.e. without thrombolytic drugs. These in vitro and in vivo experiments have confirmed this ability on several scales, ranging from tiny to large clots [10, 15, 18–23].

A recent study characterized lipid microbubble interactions with thrombi in the presence of US using an ultra-high-speed microscopy imaging system to visualize microbubble acoustic behaviors at megahertz frame rates [24]. Under inertial cavitation conditions, large-amplitude microbubble oscillations caused thrombus deformation and pitting, and acoustic radiation forces (Bjerknes forces) further augmented the microbubble-thrombus interaction.

In vivo examples of sonothrombolysis with microbubbles are almost certainly more complex, with interactions also including endothelial factors triggered by local ischemia as well as an endogenous t-PA effect originating from the ischemic vessel wall [18, 20–23]. Recently, treatment with microbubbles and US in a rabbit model of embolic stroke was shown to decrease the incidence of intracerebral hemorrhage [25] and to result in a reduction in infarct volume similar to that after t-PA treatment [26].

Targeting Sonothrombolysis with New Drug Delivery Systems
Albumin microbubbles have been tagged with the glycoprotein IIb/IIIa inhibitor ep-tifibatide to promote their accumulation at the clot for enhanced recanalization [22]. Likewise, abciximab microbubbles targeted to human platelets improve the visualization of human clots both in vitro and in an in vivo model of acute arterial thrombotic occlusion, thus demonstrating the feasibility of using a therapeutic agent for selective targeting in vascular imaging [27]. Importantly, ligand targeting of bubbles with abciximab improves the effectiveness of lysis with US [28].

Entrapment of t-PA into liposomes can also improve the efficacy of thrombolysis [29–34] through cavitational effects and acoustic radiation force [35]. Recent work suggests that t-PA-loaded, echogenic liposomes are superior to microbubbles for clot lysis by US [36]. Moreover, novel developments have combined nanotechnology with microbubbles for drug delivery [37].

Clinical Trials

The Challenge of Implementing Sonothrombolysis Through the Human Skull
Different US equipment, each with advantages and disadvantages, has been proposed for performing sonothrombolysis in stroke patients. One avenue has been to apply commercial, 2-MHz transcranial-monitoring devices to accelerate clot lysis using recombinant tissue plasminogen activator (rt-PA). Although this choice fosters rapid translation of sonothrombolysis into the clinical arena because of existing device approvals, some work has questioned whether this approach is really capable of treating ischemic stroke because of the very high attenuation of US by temporal bone [38]. In humans, this attenuation amounts to a reduction of at least 86% of the US energy of diagnostic transducers in very thin bone windows [38] and to an almost 100% reduction in patients with poor bone windows. Differences in signal absorption of the bone can lead to ten-fold differences in the mechanical index of the incident US wave [39]. The skull also greatly distorts the US field of commercial diagnostic frequencies, which causes changes in the beam area by a factor of about 4 (i.e. defocusing through phase aberration) [39]. Thus, both the local 'effective' US acoustic pressure and the treatment area delivered to any one patient for thrombolysis vary significantly, which makes comparisons of therapeutic efficacy between patients difficult. Recent computer simulations suggest that intracranial acoustic pressures achieved using diagnos-

tic devices are not high enough to enable enhancement of t-PA thrombolysis [40]. However, one may argue that the thrombolytic effect in living systems is far more complex and may be explained through an enhancing effect of US upon endogenous t-PA for clot lysis, through local renewing of plasminogen and through possible evacuation of dissolved thrombotic material by collaterals. Such hypothetical in vivo mechanisms await further substantiation.

Dedicated equipment using lower US frequencies than those of diagnostic machines is theoretically better suited for thrombolysis through the skull [41, 42] because of better penetration and superior thrombolytic effects. However, the use of lower frequencies in the skull is more complex due to potential adverse effects that do not occur at diagnostic frequencies. These effects are discussed in detail in relation to the Transcranial Low-Frequency US-Mediated Thrombolysis in Brain Ischemia (TRUMBI) trial (see below).

Trials of Ultrasound-Enhanced Thrombolysis in Ischemic Stroke
Several groups have reported the use of commercial, 2-MHz, diagnostic US devices for treating acute ischemic stroke [43–45]. The largest of these was the Combined Lysis of Thrombus in Brain Ischemia Using Transcranial US and Systemic t-PA trial [46], a multi-center, randomized clinical trial on 126 patients with acute occlusion of the middle cerebral artery (MCA). All patients were treated with intravenous rt-PA within three hours after the onset of symptoms. The target patients received 2-MHz transcranial Doppler (TCD) monitoring for two hours along with rt-PA. A complete reperfusion or dramatic clinical recovery was observed for 49% of the patients in the target group (rt-PA+US) and for only 30% of the control group. No secondary effects linked with US exposure were identified.

The TRUMBI trial used a dedicated, low-frequency, 300-kHz US device (fig. 1) for sonothrombolysis [47]. The reasons for choosing this frequency were three-fold: 1) penetration through the skull was superior to that of commercial 2-MHz probes, 2) the thrombolytic effect was faster and more efficient [42], and 3) the approach was simpler because a large volume of the brain was insonated when using low-frequency US, thus ensuring better targeting of occlusions, e.g. MCA occlusions with a variable anatomical course and branch occlusions that were not accessible to diagnostic US devices through the temporal bone window. However, the trial was stopped prematurely because of the occurrence of a higher number of intracerebral hemorrhages after t-PA treatment combined with transcranial sonication, some occurring contralateral to the ischemic lesion. Five hemorrhages in the target group were symptomatic and were possibly linked to US exposure.

The reason for the hemorrhages in the TRUMBI trial was unclear. Indeed, preclinical work in rats [48] was unable to demonstrate harmful secondary effects of US using the TRUMBI parameters. One study suggests that hemorrhages in the TRUMBI trial were related to abnormal permeability of the human blood-brain barrier that was induced by wide-field, low-frequency insonation [49]. Wang and

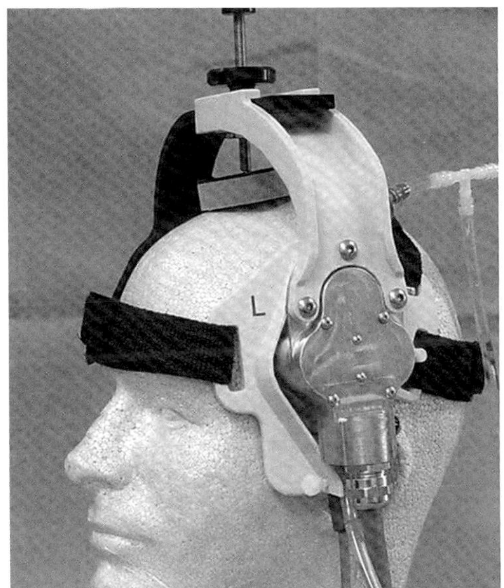 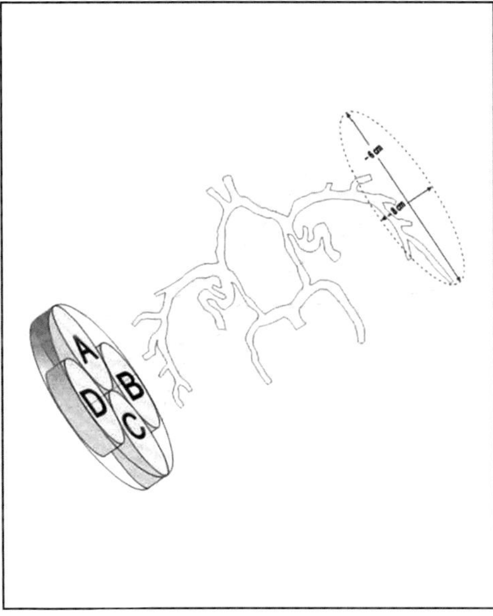

Fig. 1. The transducer has four elements (A to D) that operate in pairs to insonate a specific region of the brain. The CB pair or the CD pair treats the circle of Willis area and the M1 segment; the DB pair covers the M2 and proximal M3 segments; and the AD and AB pairs are targeted at the mid and distal M33 segments. The effective ultrasound field around the beam axis at the sonicated target area covers approximately 8 cm in the frontal-occipital direction and approximately 6 cm in the cranio-caudal direction.

coworkers hypothesized that, in the TRUMBI trial, a pulse length of 765 mm combined with a very wide beam could cause overlap many times as the wave ran its course back and forth across the brain and reflected off the skull. Therefore, the instantaneous intensity of US in the brain tissue might multiply constructively at some localized sites of brain tissue, resulting in mechanical indexes that were larger than the maximum limit set by the FDA [50]. A recent simulation of the TRUMBI trial demonstrated that pressure levels in the brain (about 0.27 MPa) were slightly above the inertial cavitation threshold, which could result in standing waves outside the targeted region [40]. Importantly, these adverse effects could be remedied through small adjustments of the US parameters in the simulation studies.

Clinical Studies Implementing Microbubble-Enhanced Thrombolysis
The first clinical trial using microbubbles in acute stroke added Levovist™ to standard t-PA therapy augmented with continuous application of TCD [51]. The outcomes were improved to a 55% sustained recanalization rate compared with a 41% rate using t-PA and continuous TCD and a 24% rate using t-PA alone. Clinical improvement was more than 4 on the NIH Stroke Scale in 55% of patients compared with 41% patients administered t-PA and continuous TCD and with 31% of patients administered t-PA alone. No increased symptomatic intracranial hemorrhage (ICH) was observed.

Another study [52] reported improved recanalization flow scores and clinical outcomes with a combined microbubble therapy using SonoVue™, while the use of perflutren lipid microbubbles showed a good safety profile with no increase in symptomatic ICH after systemic thrombolysis [53]. In an additional pilot investigation, perflutren lipid microbubbles and US were administered with t-PA to patients with proximal intracranial occlusions [54]. In patients receiving 1.4 ml of microbubbles, there were no symptomatic ICHs, whereas 27% of patients receiving 2.8 ml of microbubbles developed spontaneous intracranial hemorrhages (sICHs). Thus, two early-phase studies [53, 54] showed that, at the same dose of 1.4 ml of perflutren lipid microbubbles, no symptomatic bleeding events occurred. However, lack of knowledge of the effective intracranial acoustic pressures in individual patients makes treatment comparisons in these studies difficult.

A recent meta-analysis of all published clinical sonothrombolysis studies confirmed that US and t-PA treatment (with or without microbubbles) increases recanalization compared to t-PA treatment alone [55].

New Developments in Sonothrombolysis

Novel Operator-Independent Device for Sonothrombolysis
The Combined Lysis of Thrombus in Brain Ischemia With Transcranial Ultrasound and Systemic T-PA-Hands-Free study is a multicenter, open-label, pilot safety trial of t-PA plus a novel operator-independent US device in patients with ischemic stroke caused by proximal intracranial occlusion [56]. The device consists of a head-frame containing 18 US transducers (each operating at 2 MHz, pulsed-wave), which exposes both temporal windows and the suboccipital window. The transmission characteristics are set to emulate the acoustic characteristics of the exposure levels in the Combined Lysis of Thrombus in Brain Ischemia using Transcranial Ultrasound and Systemic t-PA trial. This new device has been well tolerated by stroke-free volunteers and did not cause any neurological dysfunction or affect blood-brain barrier integrity [56]. The first pilot studies with this device in combination with systemic t-PA have demonstrated its safety, while the recanalization rates will be evaluated in a phase-III efficacy trial [57].

MRI-Guided Focused Ultrasound for Clot Lysis
Histotripsy is a process that fractionates soft tissue through controlled cavitation using focused, short, high-intensity US pulses. Histotripsy can be used to achieve effective thrombolysis with US energy alone at peak negative acoustic pressures >6 MPa, breaking down blood clots into small fragments of less than 5 μm in diameter in about 1.5–5 minutes [58]. Recent developments in MRI-guided focused US therapy through the intact skull suggest that this technology could be useful for clot lysis in humans. Experimental studies, both for ischemic and hemorrhagic stroke, are currently being undertaken to test this possibility.

Sonothrombolysis of Spontaneous Intracranial Hemorrhages
Recently, there has been interest in the lysis of ICHs and intraventricular hemorrhages (IVHs) using catheter-mounted transducers. As compared with data from the Minimally Invasive Surgery plus T-PA for Intracerebral Hemorrhage Evacuation and Clot Lysis Evaluating Accelerated Resolution of Intraventricular Hemorrhage II studies, the rate of lysis during treatment for IVH and ICH was faster in patients treated with sonothrombolysis plus rt-PA vs. rt-PA alone [59]. Thus, lysis and drainage of spontaneous ICHs and IVHs with a reduction in the mass effect can be accomplished rapidly and safely through sonothrombolysis using stereotactically delivered drainage and US catheters via a bur hole.

Treating the Microcirculation with Ultrasound and Microbubbles
The effects of 2-MHz US and microbubbles (SonoVue™) have been studied in a permanent MCA occlusion model in rats to evaluate the possible adverse bioeffects [60] at different steps in the cascade of tissue destruction after ischemic stroke [61]. While deleterious effects were not observed, infarctions were unexpectedly smaller in the treatment group, despite the fact that recanalization of the MCA did not occur in any of the animals, suggesting a beneficial effect of US and microbubbles in the microcirculation. A similar tissue-protective effect was found in an in vivo animal study using intravenous microbubbles and transthoracic US to treat acute coronary thromboses. Pigs treated with US and intravenous perfluorocarbon-exposed sonicated dextrose albumin microbubbles had significantly greater improvements in ST segments over a 30-minute treatment period when compared with pigs treated with US alone or with control animals. Moreover, there was a significantly smaller myocardial contrast defect size after treatment with US and perfluorocarbon-exposed sonicated dextrose albumin [62]. Recently, nano-CT was used to demonstrate complete reversal of microcirculatory impairment following treatment with rt-PA, US and microbubbles in a rodent reperfusion model [63]. The mechanism of the microcirculatory effect of US and microbubbles may involve improvement of blood flow to at-risk tissue via collaterals as well as changes in the microenvironment of the damaged tissue, such as decreased cell-damaging factors, e.g. glutamate or enhanced enzyme activity of endothelial nitric oxide [64]. Further work is necessary to elucidate the exact mechanisms of salvaging at-risk tissue by US-mediated microbubble thrombolysis.

Emergency Treatment of Ischemic Stroke with Ultrasound and Microbubbles?
There has been some concern regarding possible capillary ruptures occurring during the application of US and microbubbles that might lead to increased bleeding [65]. Fortunately, this concern has been considerably reduced by work in rabbits showing that the current diagnostic US exposure levels combined with microbubbles are well below the threshold of blood-brain barrier opening or brain tissue damage [66]. One study has investigated whether US and microbubbles influence the course of intracerebral hemorrhage in a rodent model of ICH [67]. The morphometric evaluation of

hemorrhage size and brain edema after the application of US and microbubbles showed no significant effect between the treatment and control groups. Furthermore, there was no difference in apoptosis rates. This lack of an effect of US and microbubbles on cerebral hemorrhage provides the first experimental support that bleeding may not be a contraindication to treatment of ischemic stroke with this new approach. Moreover, the evidence presented above for improved flow in the microcirculation through the application of US and microcirculation suggests that this combination could be an attractive emergency adjunct treatment for ischemic stroke.

Summary

Rapid restoration of vascular flow is the primary goal of acute stroke treatment. When combined with microbubbles, US offers new thrombolytic mechanisms. Recent data suggesting that US and microbubbles can improve microvascular flow may provide new concepts for stroke treatment; however, microcirculation therapy will require new transducer designs for US delivery to this therapeutic target. Moreover, systems that estimate the intracranial acoustic pressure through direct detection of cavitation or through observations of microbubble behavior will allow more consistent application of US parameters to individual patients in clinical trials.

US-sensitive thrombolytic drug delivery combined with specific targeting is highly attractive. Targeting of clot-dissolving therapeutics could potentially decrease the frequency of complications while simultaneously increasing treatment effectiveness by concentrating the available drug at the desired site and permitting a lower systemic dose [68].

Any new system must be simple and safe when it is to be widely used. If its safety can be proven, it may be possible to use microbubble-augmented US lysis or US-augmented thrombolysis in patients who have not yet been transported to the hospital for CT imaging to determine the presence or absence of ICH, even patients who have undergone hemorrhagic strokes. Even if the improvement in outcome with this new technique is only moderate, the addition of many more patients to therapy within the earliest part of the time window would be a service with tremendous impact.

References

1 Sobbe A, Stumpff U, Trübestein G, et al: [Thrombolysis by ultrasound (author's transl)]. Klin Wochenschr 1974;52:1117–1121.

2 Harpaz D, Chen X, Francis CW, et al: Ultrasound accelerates urokinase-induced thrombolysis and reperfusion. Am Heart J 1994;127:1211–1219.

3 Rosenschein U, Gaul G, Erbel R, et al: Percutaneous transluminal therapy of occluded saphenous vein grafts: can the challenge be met with ultrasound thrombolysis? Circulation 1999;99:26–29.

4 Luo H, Birnbaum Y, Fishbein MC, et al: Enhancement of thrombolysis in vivo without skin and soft tissue damage by transcutaneous ultrasound. Thromb Res 1998;89:171–177.

5 Riggs PN, Francis CW, Bartos SR, et al: Ultrasound enhancement of rabbit femoral artery thrombolysis. Cardiovasc Surg 1997;5:201–207.

6 Hamm CW, Steffen W, Terres W, et al: Intravascular therapeutic ultrasound thrombolysis in acute myocardial infarctions. Am J Cardiol 1997;80:200–204.

7 Rosenschein U, Roth A, Rassin T, et al: Analysis of coronary ultrasound thrombolysis endpoints in acute myocardial infarction (ACUTE trial). Results of the feasibility phase. Circulation 1997;95:1411–1416.

8 Yock PG, Fitzgerald PJ: Catheter-based ultrasound thrombolysis. Circulation 1997;95:1360–1362.

9 Everbach EC, Francis CW: Cavitational mechanisms in ultrasound-accelerated thrombolysis at 1 MHz. Ultrasound Med Biol 2000;26:1153–1160.

10 Datta S, Coussios CC, McAdory LE, et al: Correlation of cavitation with ultrasound enhancement of thrombolysis. Ultrasound Med Biol 2006;32:1257–1267.

11 Siddiqi F, Odrljin TM, Fay PJ, et al: Binding of tissue-plasminogen activator to fibrin: effect of ultrasound. Blood 1998;91:2019–2025.

12 Daffertshofer M, Hennerici M: Ultrasound in the treatment of ischaemic stroke. Lancet Neurol 2003;2:283–290.

13 Tachibana K, Tachibana S: Albumin microbubble echo-contrast material as an enhancer for ultrasound accelerated thrombolysis. Circulation 1995;92:1148–1150.

14 Porter TR, LeVeen RF, Fox R, et al: Thrombolytic enhancement with perfluorocarbon-exposed sonicated dextrose albumin microbubbles. Am Heart J 1996;132:964–968.

15 Cintas P, Nguyen F, Boneu B, et al: Enhancement of enzymatic fibrinolysis with 2-MHz ultrasound and microbubbles. J Thromb Haemost 2004;2:1163–1166.

16 Datta S, Coussios CC, Ammi AY, et al: Ultrasound-enhanced thrombolysis using definity as a cavitation nucleation agent. Ultrasound Med Biol 2008;34:1421–1433.

17 Miller MW, Miller DL, Brayman AA: A review of in vitro bioeffects of inertial ultrasonic cavitation from a mechanistic perspective. Ultrasound Med Biol 1996;22:1131–1154.

18 Birnbaum Y, Luo H, Nagai T, et al: Noninvasive in vivo clot dissolution without a thrombolytic drug: recanalization of thrombosed iliofemoral arteries by transcutaneous ultrasound combined with intravenous infusion of microbubbles. Circulation 1998;97:130–134.

19 Porter TR, Kricsfeld D, Lof J, et al: Effectiveness of transcranial and transthoracic ultrasound and microbubbles in dissolving intravascular thrombi. J Ultrasound Med 2001;20:1313–1325.

20 Culp WC, Porter TR, Xie F, et al: Microbubble potentiated ultrasound as a method of declotting thrombosed dialysis grafts: experimental study in dogs. Cardiovasc Intervent Radiol 2001;24:407–412.

21 Culp WC, Erdem E, Roberson PK, et al: Microbubble potentiated ultrasound as a method of stroke therapy in a pig model: preliminary findings. J Vasc Interv Radiol 2003;14:1433–1436.

22 Culp WC, Porter TR, Lowery J, et al: Intracranial clot lysis with intravenous microbubbles and transcranial ultrasound in swine. Stroke 2004;35:2407–2411.

23 Xie F, Tsutsui JM, Lof J, et al: Effectiveness of lipid microbubbles and ultrasound in declotting thrombosis. Ultrasound Med Biol 2005;31:979–985.

24 Chen X, Leeman JE, Wang J, et al: New insights into mechanisms of sonothrombolysis using ultra-high-speed imaging. Ultrasound Med Biol 2014;40:258–262.

25 Flores R, Hennings LJ, Lowery JD, et al: Microbubble-augmented ultrasound sonothrombolysis decreases intracranial hemorrhage in a rabbit model of acute ischemic stroke. Invest Radiol 2011;46:419–424.

26 Culp WC, Flores R, Brown AT, et al: Successful microbubble sonothrombolysis without tissue-type plasminogen activator in a rabbit model of acute ischemic stroke. Stroke 2011;42:2280–2285.

27 Alonso A, Della Martina A, Stroick M, et al: Molecular imaging of human thrombus with novel abciximab immunobubbles and ultrasound. Stroke 2007;38:1508–1514.

28 Alonso A, Dempfle CE, Della Martina A, et al: In vivo clot lysis of human thrombus with intravenous abciximab immunobubbles and ultrasound. Thromb Res 2009;124:70–74.

29 Nguyen PD, O'Rear EA, Johnson AE, et al: Thrombolysis using liposomal-encapsulated streptokinase: an in vitro study. Exp Biol Med 1989;192:261–269.

30 Heeremans JL, Prevost R, Bekkers ME, et al: Thrombolytic treatment with tissue-type plasminogen activator (t-PA) containing liposomes in rabbits: a comparison with free t-PA. Thromb Haemost 1995;73:488–494.

31 Perkins WR, Vaughan DE, Plavin SR, et al: Streptokinase entrapment in interdigitation-fusion liposomes improves thrombolysis in an experimental rabbit model. Thromb Haemost 1997;77:1174–1178.

32 Leach JK, O'Rear EA, Patterson E, et al: Accelerated thrombolysis in a rabbit model of carotid artery thrombosis with liposome-encapsulated and micro-encapsulated streptokinase. Thromb Haemost 2003;90:64–70.

33 Wang SS, Chou NK, Chung TW: The t-PA-encapsulated PLGA nanoparticles shelled with CS or CS-GRGD alter both permeation through and dissolving patterns of blood clots compared with t-PA solution: an in vitro thrombolysis study. J Biomed Mater Res A 2009;91:753–761.

34 Smith DA, Vaidya SS, Kopechek JA, et al: Ultrasound-triggered release of recombinant tissue-type plasminogen activator from echogenic liposomes. Ultrasound Med Biol 2010;36:145–157.

35 Xi X, Yang F, Chen D, et al: A targeting drug-delivery model via interactions among cells and liposomes under ultrasonic excitation. Phys Med Biol 2008;53:3251–3265.

36 Laing ST, Moody MR, Kim H, et al: Thrombolytic efficacy of tissue plasminogen activator-loaded echogenic liposomes in a rabbit thrombus model. Thromb Res 2012;130:629–635.

37 Geers B, Lentacker I, Sanders NN, et al: Self-assembled liposome-loaded microbubbles: the missing link for safe and efficient ultrasound triggered drug-delivery. J Control Release 2011;152:249–256.

38 Pfaffenberger S, Devcic-Kuhar B, Kollmann C, et al: Can a commercial diagnostic ultrasound device accelerate thrombolysis? An in vitro skull model. Stroke 2005;36:124–128.

39 Hölscher T, Wilkening WG, Molkenstruck S, et al: Transcranial sound field characterization. Ultrasound Med Biol 2008;34:973–980.

40 Baron C, Aubry JF, Tanter M, et al: Simulation of intracranial acoustic fields in clinical trials of sonothrombolysis. Ultrasound Med Biol 2009;35:1148–1158.

41 Behrens S, Daffertshofer M, Spiegel D, et al: Low-frequency, low-intensity ultrasound accelerates thrombolysis through the skull. Ultrasound Med Biol 1999;25:269–273.

42 Behrens S, Spengos K, Daffertshofer M, et al: Transcranial ultrasound-improved thrombolysis: diagnostic vs. therapeutic ultrasound. Ultrasound Med Biol 2001;27:1683–1689.

43 Alexandrov AV, Demchuk AM, Felberg RA, et al: High rate of complete recanalization and dramatic clinical recovery during tPA infusion when continuously monitored with 2-MHz transcranial Doppler monitoring. Stroke 2000;31:610–614.

44 Eggers J, Koch B, Meyer K, et al: Effect of ultrasound on thrombolysis of middle cerebral artery occlusion. Ann Neurol 2003;53:797–800.

45 Cintas P, Le Traon AP, Larrue V: High rate of recanalization of middle cerebral artery occlusion during 2-MHz transcranial color-coded Doppler continuous monitoring without thrombolytic drug. Stroke 2002;33:626–628.

46 Alexandrov AV, Molina CA, Grotta JC, et al: Ultrasound-enhanced systemic thrombolysis for acute ischemic stroke. N Engl J Med 2004;351:2170–2178.

47 Daffertshofer M, Gass A, Ringleb P, et al: Transcranial low-frequency ultrasound-mediated thrombolysis in brain ischemia: increased risk of hemorrhage with combined ultrasound and tissue plasminogen activator: results of a phase II clinical trial. Stroke 2005;36:1441–1446.

48 Daffertshofer M, Huang Z, Fatar M, et al: Efficacy of sonothrombolysis in a rat model of embolic ischemic stroke. Neurosci Lett 2004;361:115–119.

49 Reinhard M, Hetzel A, Krüger S, et al: Blood-brain barrier disruption by low-frequency ultrasound. Stroke 2006;37:1546–1548.

50 Wang Z, Moehring MA, Voie AH, et al: In vitro evaluation of dual mode ultrasonic thrombolysis method for transcranial application with an occlusive thrombosis model. Ultrasound Med Biol 2008;34:96–102.

51 Molina CA, Ribo M, Rubiera M, et al: Microbubble administration accelerates clot lysis during continuous 2-MHz ultrasound monitoring in stroke patients treated with intravenous tissue plasminogen activator. Stroke 2006;37:425–429.

52 Perren F, Loulidi J, Poglia D, et al: Microbubble potentiated transcranial duplex ultrasound enhances IV thrombolysis in acute stroke. J Thromb Thrombolysis 2008;25:219–223.

53 Alexandrov AV, Mikulik R, Ribo M, et al: A pilot randomized clinical safety study of sonothrombolysis augmentation with ultrasound-activated perflutren-lipid microspheres for acute ischemic stroke. Stroke 2008;39:1464–1469.

54 Molina CA, Barreto AD, Tsivgoulis G, et al: Transcranial ultrasound in clinical sonothrombolysis (TUCSON) trial. Ann Neurol 2009;66:28–38.

55 Tsivgoulis G, Eggers J, Ribo M, et al: Safety and efficacy of ultrasound-enhanced thrombolysis: a comprehensive review and meta-analysis of randomized and nonrandomized studies. Stroke 2010;41:280–287.

56 Barlinn K, Barreto AD, Sisson A, et al: CLOTBUST-hands Free: initial safety testing of a novel operator-independent ultrasound device in stroke-free volunteers. Stroke 2013;44:1641–1646.

57 Barreto AD, Alexandrov AV, Shen L, et al: CLOTBUST-hands Free: pilot safety study of a novel operator-independent ultrasound device in patients with acute ischemic stroke. Stroke 2013;44:3376–3381.

58 Maxwell AD, Cain CA, Duryea AP, et al: Noninvasive thrombolysis using pulsed ultrasound cavitation therapy – histotripsy. Ultrasound Med Biol 2009;35:1982–1994.

59 Newell DW, Shah MM, Wilcox R, et al: Minimally invasive evacuation of spontaneous intracerebral hemorrhage using sonothrombolysis. J Neurosurg 2011;115:592–601.

60 Fatar M, Stroick M, Griebe M, et al: Effect of combined ultrasound and microbubbles treatment in an experimental model of cerebral ischemia. Ultrasound Med Biol 2008;34:1414–1420.

61 Dirnagl U, Iadecola C, Moskowitz MA: Pathobiology of ischaemic stroke: an integrated view. Trends Neurosci 1999;22:391–397.

62 Xie F, Slikkerveer J, Gao S, et al: Coronary and micro-vascular thrombolysis with guided diagnostic ultrasound and microbubbles in acute ST segment elevation myocardial infarction. J Am Soc Echocardiogr 2011;24:1400–1408.

63 Nedelmann M, Ritschel N, Doenges S, et al: Combined contrast-enhanced ultrasound and rt-PA treatment is safe and improves impaired microcirculation after reperfusion of middle cerebral artery occlusion. J Cereb Blood Flow Metab 2010;30:1712–1720.

64 Altland OD, Dalecki D, Suchkova VN, et al: Low-intensity ultrasound increases endothelial cell nitric oxide synthase activity and nitric oxide synthesis. J Thromb Haemost 2004;2:637–643.

65 Skyba DM, Price RJ, Linka AZ, et al: Direct in vivo visualization of intravascular destruction of microbubbles by ultrasound and its local effects on tissue. Circulation 1998;98:290–293.

66 Hynynen K, McDannold N, Martin H, et al: The threshold for brain damage in rabbits induced by bursts of ultrasound in the presence of an ultrasound contrast agent (Optison). Ultrasound Med Biol 2003;29:473–481.

67 Stroick M, Alonso A, Fatar M, et al: Effects of simultaneous application of ultrasound and microbubbles on intracerebral hemorrhage in an animal model. Ultrasound Med Biol 2006;32:1377–1382.

68 Marsh JN, Senpan A, Hu G, et al: Fibrin-targeted perfluorocarbon nanoparticles for targeted thrombolysis. Nanomedicine-UK 2007;2:533–543.

Prof. Stephen Meairs, MD, PhD
Department of Neurology
Universitätsmedizin Mannheim, University of Heidelberg
Theodor-Kutzer-Ufer 1–3, DE–68167 Mannheim (Germany)
E-Mail meairs@neuro.ma.uni-heidelberg.de

Alonso A, Hennerici MG, Meairs S (eds): Translational Neurosonology.
Front Neurol Neurosci. Basel, Karger, 2015, vol 36, pp 94–105 (DOI: 10.1159/000366241)

Non-Invasive Transcranial Brain Ablation with High-Intensity Focused Ultrasound

Jürgen W. Jenne

Fraunhofer MEVIS, Institute for Medical Image Computing, Bremen, Germany

Abstract

The idea to ablate brain tissue with high-intensity focused ultrasound (HIFU) in a highly precise and localized manner is relatively old. For HIFU tissue ablation, ultrasound (US) waves are concentrated to a focal point. Due to US absorption, the focal area will be heated and consequently thermally destroyed. The spatial accuracy of the non-invasive procedure and the sharp delineation of the induced tissue lesions have led to the term 'focused ultrasound surgery' (FUS). The major obstacle for HIFU ablation in the brain is the skull bone, which absorbs most of the US energy and disturbs the focused US field. The development of large-sized phased array US transducers and adaptive focusing techniques based on computed tomography images have allowed these difficulties to be overcome. With the combination of FUS and MR-imaging and MR-thermometry (MR-guided Focused Ultrasound Surgery, MRgFUS), real-time therapy guidance and control has been established. The safety, feasibility and effectiveness of transcranial MRgFUS were investigated in four initial clinical studies including 4 to 15 patients each. In the first study, which dealt with the treatment of inoperable recurrent glioblastoma, MR was used to monitor localized tissue heating, but no tissue ablation was possible due to technical restrictions of the treatment setup. With improved equipment, the precise induction of thermal lesions in the target area was achieved in studies on neuropathic pain and essential tremor. An instantaneous and persistent significant improvement of disease symptoms was observed in most patients. However, there were serious adverse effects in two cases, where intracranial hemorrhages appeared due to the induction of cavitation. Based on these encouraging clinical results, more extensive clinical studies have been initiated. Transcranial MRgFUS is a fast-growing field of neurological research with high clinical potential.

Introduction

The clinical application of high-intensity focused ultrasound (HIFU) for thermal tissue ablation, also called focused ultrasound surgery (FUS) due to its precision, has been around for some time. Indeed, the idea for localized brain therapy gave the impetus for the early development of the HIFU technology. In 1942, Lynn et al. treated animal brains and found well-demarcated tissue necrosis [1, 2]. Later, starting in the 50s, William and Francis Fry investigated HIFU therapy to induce functional changes in the central nervous system [3]. Over time, considerable important technical developments were achieved, resulting in a number of clinical studies of HIFU for the treatment of diverse brain diseases. However, these studies had varying success due to several reasons. Some major disadvantages included the necessity of creating an acoustic window by removing parts of the skull as well as the lack of adequate imaging methods for exact treatment planning and therapy control [4]. In addition, with the progress and dissemination of radiation therapy, the clinical interest in and intensity of research on HIFU has decreased notably.

Due to the introduction of new imaging methods, in particular, diagnostic ultrasound (US) and magnetic resonance imaging (MRI), there has been increasing interest in HIFU therapies during the past 20 years. Two steps were crucial for the development of transcranial applications. The development of large-scale, phased array therapeutic US transducers [5, 6] allowed application of HIFU through the intact skull. In addition, MRI, with its unique attribute of *non-invasive* tissue thermometry, gave a major impetus for further development of HIFU for brain therapy.

Beside focal brain tissue ablation, transcranial-focused US offers additional approaches for therapeutic use in the neurological field. In combination with the administration of microbubbles, focused US at moderate power levels can locally and reversibly open the blood-brain barrier, e.g. to enhance drug delivery. Another proposed therapy approach is US-mediated lysis of blood clots to treat ischemic stroke.

This article focuses on tissue ablation therapy, in particular, under MRI online control, i.e. MRgFUS. Both blood-brain barrier opening and sonothrombolysis are discussed in separate articles in this book.

Ultrasound Tissue Interaction

To understand the therapeutic potential of US and its related technical and biological challenges, it is important to consider the basic US-tissue interaction mechanisms. When a US wave propagates through biological tissue, thermal and mechanical, or non-thermal, effects occur. The major thermal effect is US absorption, which is the transformation of acoustic energy to heat. Absorption of US leads to tissue heating and, at high US intensities, to thermal tissue destruction due to protein coagulation [7]. It is important for cranial applications that bony structures, e.g. the skull, have a much higher absorption (30–60 times) and, accordingly, higher attenuation than soft brain tissue.

The major non-thermal US effect is cavitation. Acoustic cavitation is the formation and dynamic behavior of cavities and microbubbles in a US field. Due to high negative-pressure amplitudes, fluids can break up, and cavitation bubbles will arise. These bubbles oscillate in the US field (stable cavitation) and can grow rapidly and collapse wildly (inertial cavitation). Both, stable and inertial cavitation can cause various biological effects. For example, bubble oscillation and collapse can increase cell membrane permeability for drugs (sonoporation), which can be used for enhanced drug delivery (see 'Ultrasound-Induced Blood-Brain Barrier Opening for Drug Delivery' by A. Alonso). Cavitation activity also has the potential to destroy cells and cause bleeding (see 'Ultrasound Bioeffects and Safety Considerations' by G. ter Haar). The occurrence of cavitation is a threshold phenomenon that depends on various parameters. High rarefaction pressure, low frequency and, in particular, the presence of synthetic microbubbles, e.g. US contrast agent, increase the probability of the occurrence of cavitation.

Additional mechanical US effects include a permanent radiation pressure when the momentum of the absorbed US field is transferred to the propagated tissue and, consequently, steady radiation force and acoustic streaming. Such fluid-mechanical effects are thought to be the basic mechanisms for targeted stimulation of neuronal activities [8, 9]. With an adequate choice of US parameters (frequency, pressure, pulse duration, exposure time, etc.), one can selectively emphasize one US effect or another. For instance, thermal tissue ablation uses long pulses (on the order of seconds) at moderate pressure levels (~10 MPa). However, the other effects cannot always be suppressed completely, which can cause side effects.

High-Intensity Focused Ultrasound and Magnetic Resonance-Guided Focused Ultrasound Surgery: Basics and Principles

The principle of HIFU tissue ablation (FUS) is rather simple. A piezoelectric transducer generates a focused US field that is transmitted through the intact skin and deep into the tissue. Due to the high-intensity US, the tissue at the focal point heats up within seconds, the cells are thermally destroyed, and sharply demarcated tissue necrosis occurs. Depending on the focal length and the aperture of the transducer, single lesions are rather small. To ablate larger areas, multiple single lesions are combined into a contiguous region of necrosis (spot-scanning technique). However, a sufficient pause time between single sonications is necessary to prevent tissue overheating, boiling and bubble formation, which could lead to unpredictable lesion growth [10]. To ablate large target volumes, e.g. an extended tumor, very long treatment times can be required.

Nevertheless, the *non-invasive* ablation of brain tissue through the intact skull by HIFU imposes much higher demands, as the skull bone absorbs most of the insonated US energy. On the one hand, this treatment can lead to an unwanted and potentially harmful temperature elevation of the cranial bone. On the other hand, the applied total energy has to be sufficiently high so that enough energy passes the skull for localized focal tissue ablation.

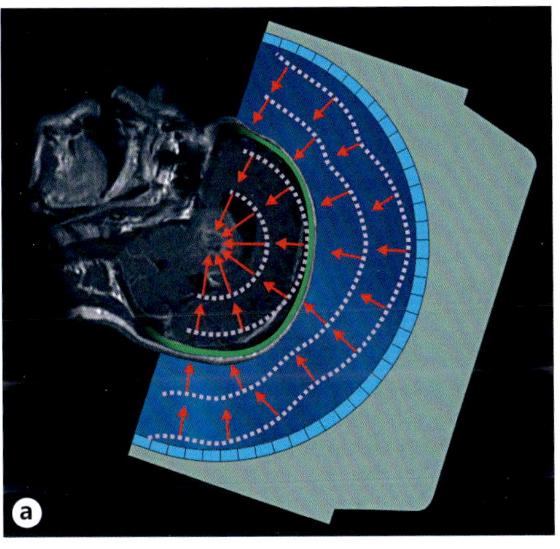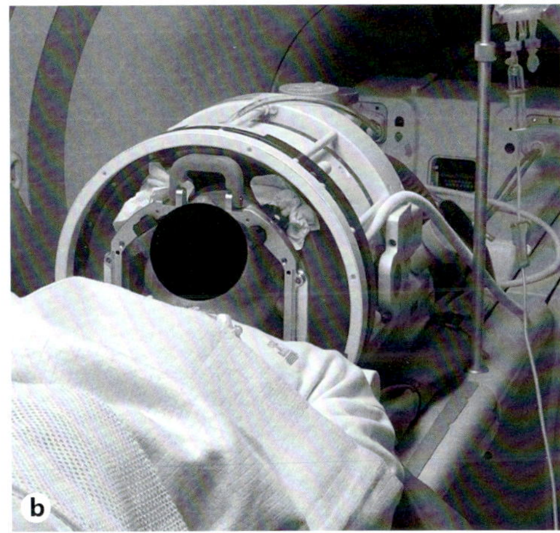

Fig. 1. a Schematic illustration of transcranial FUS ablation. A helmet-like phased array transducer (light blue) generates a focused ultrasound field in the brain. Degassed water (dark blue) between the transducer and the skull bone ensures US coupling and bone cooling. The dashed lines illustrate the phase-corrected US field. **b** Photograph of the treatment setup. The patient is positioned on the MR table, with the head fixed in the therapy helmet by a stereotactic frame (Courtesy: InSightec LTD, Tirat Carmel, Israel, illustration (**a**), and Center for MR-Research, University Children's Hospital Zurich, Switzerland, photo (**b**)).

In addition, the skull is shaped irregularly and has variable thickness and acoustic impedance, which leads to distortion of the penetrating US waves. Thus, an accurately focused US field will lose its focused character and the targeted position by passing the skull bones.

To overcome these difficulties, large-scale, hemispherical transducers that cover a major part of the skull and consist of up to one thousand array elements were developed [5, 11]. Due to the large area of the transducer, the acoustic energy is spread all over the skull. Hence, the energy density and, subsequently, the heating of the bone are minimized. In addition, the coupling fluid, i.e. degassed water, between the transducer and the head surface actively cools the cranial bone. Despite the high number of phased array elements, every element can be driven with a different phase and intensity, which enables wave-distortion compensation due to the cranial bone. In the therapy-planning process, adaptive focusing methods are necessary to calculate the adequate treatment parameters for individual skull geometry, which is assessed by computed tomography (CT) (fig. 1) [6, 12].

Beside the ability to accurately focus the US through the skull bone, the use of a suitable diagnostic and image therapy-guiding tool is a necessary prerequisite for precise and safe US ablation therapy. For brain treatment, MRI is by far the best-suited imaging modality, and MRI therefore plays a crucial role in brain therapy. With its high soft-tissue contrast, MRI provides the required diagnostic information for therapy planning, i.e. precise target definition and segmentation. The second fa-

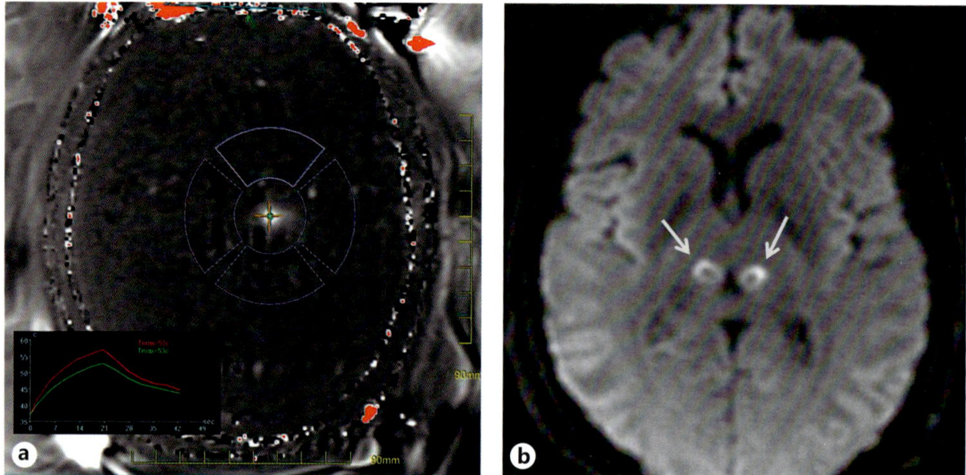

Fig. 2. a MR Thermometry. Phase image at the end of the sonication pulse. The bright area indicates the thermal spot (yellow cross). Insert: Temporal temperature development. The red curve shows the temperature development at the hottest point (one pixel), and the green curve is an averaged temperature value around this pixel. **b** Diffusion tensor image after bilateral central lateral thalamotomies. The ablated areas are clearly visible (arrows) (Courtesy: Center for MR-Research, University Children's Hospital Zurich, Switzerland).

vorable characteristic of MRI is its ability to assess the tissue temperature with MR thermometry. Several MR parameters are sensitive to temperature change, e.g. T1- and T2-relaxation times, proton resonance shift, diffusion etc. An excellent review on MR-thermometry is given by V. Rieke and K. Butts Pauly [13]. Today, the proton resonance shift method has given the best results for temperature monitoring and is used in all actual studies (fig. 2). MR temperature data acquisition starts before and ends after US application to get reference images before and to observe the cooling process after the US pulse. This technique allows calculation of the applied thermal dose and, consequently, an estimation of the destroyed tissue area [14]. Furthermore, the assessment of the temperature of critical structures, such as the skull, the dura or organs at risk, is possible. In addition, MR thermometry enables the detection of pre-therapeutic test pulses. These low-intensity US pulses heat the tissue in the focal zone to a few degrees below the threshold of ablation and serve as a control for the planed focus position.

Another promising approach, although not yet in clinical use, is MR acoustic radiation force imaging (MR-ARFI). For MR-ARFI, short US pulses are applied to the tissue. Due to the radiation force of the US field (see above), the tissue in the focal zone is moved. This small induced tissue displacement is measured by MRI, which has a resolution of micrometers [15] and allows for not only the detection of the actual US focus position without significant tissue heating but also an estimation of the acoustic beam intensity at the target [16]. This information can also be used to compensate for skull distortion [17]. Recently, Marsac et al. showed ex vivo that MR-ARFI-optimized skull aberration correction was more favorable than CT-based methods [18].

Last but not least, at the end of HIFU therapy, MRI can be used to detect the HIFU-induced tissue changes to assess the first-treatment outcome. Beside high-resolution, morphological T1w and T2w sequences, diffusion tensor imaging is used to show the induced lesions and the development of the typical edema in the treated area (fig. 2). However, contrast-enhanced T1w images, which are also used in abdominal HIFU ablations and indicate the full perfusion stop in the ablated tissue and the surrounding hyperemic rim [19], seems not to be necessary in brain applications.

Transcranial Magnetic Resonance-Guided Focused Ultrasound Surgery Therapy Systems

The use of MR guidance increases the requirements of the HIFU/MRgFUS therapy unit. This unit must be compatible with MRI, which means that neither the MR imaging may be influenced by the HIFU-system nor the MR scanner may influence the HIFU system. Furthermore, all components, e.g. the large hemispheric transducer or the stereotactic framework, have to be integrated in the limited space of the magnet bore. Today, two companies have developed MRgFUS setups for transcranial brain therapy. All clinical studies were performed with the commercially available ExAblate systems (ExAblate 3000/4000/Neuro) that were developed and manufactured by In-Sightec LTD (Tirat Carmel, Israel). The ExAblate Neuro system uses a hemispheric, i.e. helmet-like, phased array US transducer with 1,024 single elements (fig. 1) and operates at a frequency of 650 kHz, but is only available for GE MRI scanners (GE Healthcare, Milwaukee, WI, USA). After studies on animals, primates and cadavers, the first clinical safety and feasibility studies were completed. SuperSonic Imagine (SSI, Aix-en-Provence, France) also developed a transcranial MRgFUS system for clinical use. This system operates at 1 MHz with a 512-element transducer. The system is currently being tested in pre-clinical research.

Even though the treated diseases are diverse, the therapy course for transcranial HIFU ablation under MRI guidance is similar. The important steps are listed:
- The patient's head is shaved to enable good acoustic coupling.
- The head is fixed in a stereotactic frame (fig. 1).
- Adequate MRI diagnostics for treatment planning are performed.
- High-resolution CT images for skull-induced beam aberration correction are obtained.
- Therapy planning is performed.
- The target region and at-risk organs are defined. The US treatment parameters and the necessary phase correction are calculated. For tumor ablation, the target definition is based on MR diagnostics. For functional neurosurgery, atlas data are used.

- The patient's head is fixed in the therapy transducer.
- A tight circular membrane around the head is used to contain the coupling and cooling fluid (degassed and chilled water) between the skull and the transducer bowl. Patients are sedated but remain awake to enable communication and examination by the therapist.
- Accurate US-focusing with sub-therapeutic test pulses are applied under MR-thermometry control.
- Single ablation pulses are applied.
- MRI thermometry allows for stopping the US exposure at a predefined maximum temperature (fig. 2). In addition, a cavitation detector stops energy delivery immediately when cavitation occurs.
- The patient is examined to assess the result after each single sonication by the therapist.
- An adequate pause time between the single sonications is used to prevent excessive heating.
- At the end of the therapy, MR imaging for lesion detection and assessment of the first outcome is performed (fig. 2).

Clinical Studies

As indicated, there have been only a few clinical attempts to use HIFU for brain ablation [20–22]. The first clinical trial to treat brain tumors with transcranial MRgFUS was performed by a group at Brigham and Women's Hospital in Boston, MA, which had one of the leading roles in the development of MRgFUS [23]. This group treated three patients with inoperable recurrent glioblastoma; the tumors were deep-seated and centrally located in the brain. The major aim of the study was to test the feasibility and safety of the therapy procedure. The group used the ExAbalte 3000 (512 elements, 670 kHz frequency, 650–800 W total power) in a 1.5T GE MRI scanner. The skull bone heating during the ablation process was measured apart from the temperature in the focal area; however, it was not possible to observe the focal heating in all single sonications. As sufficient power was not available, the maximum induced focal temperature was only 42–51 °C after a 20-s sonication. In line with this value, no thermal lesions were detected. The maximum temperature increase in the skull was calculated to be 3.8 °C at a distance of 7 mm from the brain surface. As one patient reported sonication-related pain, the maximum applied US power was reduced. In these three patients, no other side effects, such as skin burns or skin pain, were found. Although the goal of transcranially ablating brain tissue with MRgFUS was not fully achieved, the selected data allowed interpolation of the necessary US parameters for brain tissue ablation. Based on these data, the treatment setup was improved. Using the ExAblate 4000, the number of elements was doubled, the maximum power was increased, and the US frequency was lowered.

However, the study was halted when a fourth patient died due to a cavitation-induced intracranial hemorrhage [24]. As a consequence, a detector that monitors and stops the sonication if cavitation events are detected was introduced.

The first transcranial MRgFUS for *non-invasive* functional neurosurgery was performed at the University Children's Hospital in Zurich, Switzerland [25, 26]. The aim of this study was *non-invasive*, central lateral thalamotomies as a treatment for therapy-resistant, chronic neuropathic pain. The therapy was performed using an ExAblate 4000 system in a 3T MR-scanner.

Thermally ablated lesions were induced in the posterior part of the central lateral thalamic nucleus in 11 patients. The maximum induced temperature was 51–64°C during a 10–20 s total insonation time and up to 1200 W acoustic power. The induced lesions, which were best visible on T2w and diffusion tensor images 2 days after treatment, had an ellipsoid shape with a diameter of about 3–4 mm and a length of 4–5 mm (19 lesions in 9 patients). The lesions were surrounded by a vasogenic edema. However, lesion detection was not possible in the first two patients. Pain assessment by means of a detailed questionnaire and VAS rating of pain intensity was performed in 9 patients. Six patients felt instantaneous pain relief during or at the end of the therapy. The mean pain relief after 2 days, 3 months and 1 year was found to be 71% (9 patients), 49% (9 patients) and 60% (8 patients), respectively. The VAS pain intensity scores before therapy and at 3-month and 1-year follow-up were approximately 60, 34 and 35, respectively. In addition, quantitative electroencephalography showed a significant reduction of over-activities. In one patient, bleeding appeared (8–10-mm diameter) in the targeted region, causing a dysmetria that disappeared after 1 year, except for the finer functions of speaking and writing. Other significant treatment-related adverse effects were not reported.

Two clinical studies for the treatment of movement disorder were performed. Both focused on transcranial MRgFUS thalamotomy for the treatment of essential tremor (ET).

Lipsman et al. from Toronto, Canada presented a proof-of-concept study with 4 patients with chronic and medication-resistant ET [27]. The experiments were performed using the ExAblate Neuro device in a 3T GE MR scanner. First, test pulses were used to verify the assumed focus position at the VIM nucleus. Then, a small focal lesion that was expected to have transient and reversible effects was created. The lesion was enlarged in a stepwise manner by means of increasing either the temperature (0, 1, 2°C) or the exposure duration (10–25 s). After each sonication, the lesion size and the clinical effects were assessed, and this was continued until tremor suppression or an adverse effect (e.g. paresthesia) was detected. In the case of an adverse effect, the position of the beam was corrected. In all cases, the first benefits occurred at a temperature of 50°C, and each consecutive sonication reduced the tremor. The procedure was continued until the tremor was completely stopped. The necessary number of sonications varied from 12 to 29, and the duration of the whole therapy procedure was 5–6 h.

After 1 and 3 months, the reduction in the tremor in the targeted dominant arm of the patients was found to be 89 and 81% on the clinical rating scale for tremor, respectively, and motor-task impairments were reduced by 46 and 40%, respectively. The authors reported that all patients were able to write their name and drink from a cup without help, which was not possible for them before the therapy.

In two cases, paresthesias developed during the ablation process. In one case, the paresthesia persisted in the tips of the thumb and the index finger at the 3-month follow-up. In another patient, deep vein thrombosis in the lower limb, possibly due to the length of the procedure, developed after approximately 1 week. Other side effects were not reported. In addition, the authors compared the HIFU- and radiofrequency-induced lesions and found similar radiological presentations. Based on this finding, they expected similar long-term results and adverse effects for both methods.

At the University of Virginia in Charlottesville, a larger pilot study with a 12-month follow-up was performed. This group also performed unilateral transcranial MRgFUS thalamotomy for medication refractory ET in 15 patients [28]. The aim of this preliminary study was to assess the safety, feasibility and effectiveness of tremor suppression as well as the change in the patients' quality of life. The group also used the ExAblate Neuro system in a 3T GE MR-scanner. The therapy procedure was comparable to the trial in Toronto, but with a closer follow-up of 1 day, 1 week and 1, 3 and 12 months and a deeper data analysis. Tremor in the contralateral/dominant hand, as measured on the clinical rating scale for tremor, significantly ($p = 0.001$) decreased by about 79 and 75% 3 and 12 months after therapy, respectively. The total tremor score after 12 months improved by about 56% ($p = 0.001$), while no significant ($p = 0.9$) change was seen in the ipsilateral hand. After 1 year, the relative reduction in functional disability was 85% ($p = 0.001$). The patients' perception of their quality of life improved from 37 to 12% ($p = 0.001$), and physical performance, e.g. eating, significantly improved in all patients. The authors give a detailed analysis of the adverse events that occurred during therapy and follow-up. Related to thalamotomy, the only serious adverse event was a persistent dysesthesia in the index finger in one patient over 12 months. Paresthesias of the lip, tongue and finger were the most common side effects and were mostly transient. However, chronic paresthesia was found in 4 patients after 12 months. Other transient events included a feeling of unsteadiness, ataxia, dysmetria, weak grip and slurred speech. The sonication-related transient side effects included head pain, sensations such as 'warm', 'falling' and 'spinning', light-headedness and nausea. Other side effects were related to the use of the stereotactic frame and MR imaging.

MR imaging was performed for radiological assessment after therapy. Acute lesions were visible on T2w and diffusion-weighted images. In addition, after 24 h and 1 week, a perilesional vasogenic edema was detected on T2w and FLAIR (fluid-attenuated inversion recovery) images, which resolved after 1 month. After 3 months, lesions were hardly detectable in all cases, and hemorrhage did not occur. However, susceptibility-weighted imaging showed a hypo-intense signal throughout the study that should be interpreted as degraded blood products.

In two of the above-described patient studies, the accuracy of transcranial MRgFUS was analyzed. Moser et al. used MR imaging and a stereotactic atlas of the human thalamus and basal ganglia to assess the global target accuracy in 9 MRgFUS procedures for transcranial functional neurosurgery. This group found the global target accuracy to be 0.54–0.72 mm, with 85% of the measured coordinates within a distance of 1 mm [29]. Through procedural changes, it was possible to further improve this accuracy [25].

Based on these encouraging therapy results, several clinical studies were designed and initiated. For ET therapy, a phase-III, double-blinded, multi-center, randomized study is underway (http://www.clinicaltrials.gov/ct2/show/study/NCT01827904?term=NCT01827904). A phase-I study for tremor-dominant Parkinson's disease is being performed at the University of Virginia (http://www.clinicaltrials.gov/ct2/show/record/NCT01772693?term=transcranial+ultrasound++Insightec&rank=2). In addition, other diseases have been proposed for therapy with transcranial MRgFUS ablation, e.g. epilepsy or trigeminal neuralgia, as well as cingulotomy for psychiatric disorders [30].

Conclusions and Perspectives

Transcranial MR-guided FUS is a new kind of neurosurgery that enables completely *non-invasive*, localized brain tissue ablation without opening the skull. Aside from its *non-invasive* character, the list of advantages of this method is long. Due to the small size of the single-induced tissue lesion, the generation of nearly any lesion shape is possible. HIFU ablation causes an instantaneous treatment effect, especially when compared to radiation therapy. Moreover, the treatment is free of ionizing radiation and is repeatable. The possibly most valuable advantage is the immediate feedback that is given by quasi-real-time MR guidance to control the lesion position and the thermal tissue ablation process by assessing the thermal dose.

In the future, the combination of localized US neurostimulation with MRgFUS ablation could be of particular interest. Focused, low-intensity US exposure has been shown to stimulate neuronal activity in the brain without noticeable tissue damage.

However, transcranial MRgFUS also has its limitations. The treatment time is rather long, especially for the ablation of a large target volume, e.g. an extended tumor. Due to the physically unfavorable situation arising from the US-absorbing and field-disturbing skull, safe ablation near the cranial bone is not currently possible. Moreover, the long treatment time and the high technical effort make the therapy expensive.

Whether the clinical results are worth this effort must be answered in further clinical trials. MRgFUS for brain therapy is a very active and exciting research topic. It is clear that the potential of transcranial MRgFUS has not yet been sufficiently exploited, and further clinical, preclinical and technical developments are necessary.

Acknowledgements

The author thanks Beat Werner, University Children's Hospital Zurich and InSightec LTD, Tirat Carmel for the provision of images. Thanks to Julia Schwaab, mediri GmbH, for her help in preparing the manuscript.

References

1 Lynn JG, Zwemer RL, Chick AJ, et al: A new method for the generation and use of focused ultrasound in experimental biology. J Gen Physiol 1942;26:179–193.

2 Lynn JG, Putnam TJ: Histology of cerebral lesions produced by focused ultrasound. Am J Pathol 1944;20:637–649.

3 Fry WJ, Barnard JW, Fry EJ, et al: Ultrasonic lesions in the mammalian central nervous system. Science 1955;122:517–518.

4 Jagannathan J, Sanghvi NT, Crum LA, et al: High-intensity focused ultrasound surgery of the brain: part 1 – a historical perspective with modern applications. Neurosurgery 2009;64:201–210.

5 Hynynen K, McDannold N, Clement G, et al: Preclinical testing of a phased array ultrasound system for MRI-guided noninvasive surgery of the brain – a primate study. Eur J Radiol 2006;59:149–156.

6 Aubry JF, Tanter M, Pernot M, et al: Experimental demonstration of noninvasive transskull adaptive focusing based on prior computed tomography scans. J Acoust Soc Am 2003;113:84–93.

7 Hill CR, Rivens I, Vaughan MG, et al: Lesion development in focused ultrasound surgery: a general model. Ultrasound Med Biol 1994;20:259–269.

8 Tufail Y, Matyushov A, Baldwin N, et al: Transcranial pulsed ultrasound stimulates intact brain circuits. Neuron 2010;66:681–694.

9 Tyler WJ: Noninvasive neuromodulation with ultrasound? A continuum mechanics hypothesis. Neuroscientist 2011;17:25–36.

10 Khokhlova VA, Bailey MR, Reed JA, et al: Effects of nonlinear propagation, cavitation, and boiling in lesion formation by high intensity focused ultrasound in a gel phantom. J Acoust Soc Am 2006;119:1834–1848.

11 Pernot M, Aubry JF, Tanter M, et al: High power transcranial beam steering for ultrasonic brain therapy. Phys Med Biol 2003;48:2577–2589.

12 Clement GT, Hynynen K: A non-invasive method for focusing ultrasound through the human skull. Phys Med Biol 2002;47:1219–1236.

13 Rieke V, Pauly KB: MR thermometry. J Magn Reson Im 2008;27:376–390.

14 Chung AH, Jolesz FA, Hynynen K: Thermal dosimetry of a focused ultrasound beam in vivo by magnetic resonance imaging. Med Phys 1999;26:2017–2026.

15 McDannold N, Maier SE: Magnetic resonance acoustic radiation force imaging. Med Phys 2008;35:3748–3758.

16 Paquin R, Vignaud A, Marsac L, et al: Keyhole acceleration for magnetic resonance acoustic radiation force imaging (mr arfi). Magn Reson Imaging 2013;31:1695–1703.

17 Hertzberg Y, Volovick A, Zur Y, et al: Ultrasound focusing using magnetic resonance acoustic radiation force imaging: application to ultrasound transcranial therapy. Med Phys 2010;37:2934–2942.

18 Marsac L, Chauvet D, Larrat B, et al: MR-guided adaptive focusing of therapeutic ultrasound beams in the human head. Med Phys 2012;39:1141–1149.

19 Huber PE, Jenne JW, Rastert R, et al: A new noninvasive approach in breast cancer therapy using magnetic resonance imaging-guided focused ultrasound surgery. Cancer Res 2001;61:8441–8447.

20 Heimburger RF: Ultrasound augmentation of central nervous system tumor therapy. Indiana Med 1985;78:469–476.

21 Hickey RC, Fry WJ, Meyers R, et al: Human pituitary irradiation with focused ultrasound. An initial report on effect in advanced breast cancer. Arch Surg 1961;83:620–633.

22 Ram Z, Cohen ZR, Harnof S, et al: Magnetic resonance imaging-guided, high-intensity focused ultrasound for brain tumor therapy. Neurosurgery 2006;59:949–955.

23 McDannold N, Clement GT, Black P, et al: Transcranial magnetic resonance imaging- guided focused ultrasound surgery of brain tumors: initial findings in 3 patients. Neurosurgery 2010;66:323–332.

24 Medel R, Monteith SJ, Elias WJ, et al: Magnetic resonance-guided focused ultrasound surgery: part 2: A review of current and future applications. Neurosurgery 2012;71:755–763.

25 Jeanmonod D, Werner B, Morel A, et al: Transcranial magnetic resonance imaging-guided focused ultrasound: noninvasive central lateral thalamotomy for chronic neuropathic pain. Neurosurg Focus 2012;32:E1.

26 Martin E, Jeanmonod D, Morel A, et al: High-intensity focused ultrasound for noninvasive functional neurosurgery. Ann Neurol 2009;66:858–861.

27 Lipsman N, Schwartz ML, Huang Y, et al: MR-guided focused ultrasound thalamotomy for essential tremor: A proof-of-concept study. Lancet Neurol 2013;12:462–468.

28 Elias WJ, Huss D, Voss T, et al: A pilot study of focused ultrasound thalamotomy for essential tremor. N Engl J Med 2013;369:640–648.

29 Moser D, Zadicario E, Schiff G, et al: Measurement of targeting accuracy in focused ultrasound functional neurosurgery. Neurosurg Focus 2012;32:E2.

30 Monteith S, Sheehan J, Medel R, et al: Potential intracranial applications of magnetic resonance-guided focused ultrasound surgery. J Neurosurg 2013;118:215–221.

Dr.rer.nat. Jürgen W. Jenne
Fraunhofer MEVIS
Institute for Medical Image Computing
Universitätsallee 29, DE–28359 Bremen (Germany)
E-Mail juergen.jenne@mevis.fraunhofer.de

Alonso A, Hennerici MG, Meairs S (eds): Translational Neurosonology.
Front Neurol Neurosci. Basel, Karger, 2015, vol 36, pp 106–115 (DOI: 10.1159/000366242)

Ultrasound-Induced Blood-Brain Barrier Opening for Drug Delivery

Angelika Alonso

Department of Neurology, Universitätsmedizin Mannheim, University of Heidelberg, Mannheim, Germany

Abstract

Treatment of central nervous system (CNS) diseases is highly limited due to the presence of the blood-brain barrier (BBB), which prevents the entry of approximately 99% of potential therapeutic agents into the CNS. Focused ultrasound (FUS) in combination with microbubbles can lead to a transient and focal opening of the BBB, thus enabling the passage of therapeutic agents across the BBB. Mechanical ultrasound effects, such as stable and inertial cavitation, contribute to BBB opening, possibly via transient disintegration of tight junctions. Facilitation of transcellular passage through vesicle transport may also be influenced. FUS-induced BBB opening can be performed without tissue damage, given an optimal set of ultrasound parameters. However, the risk of parenchymal damage or microhaemorrhage increases with increasing acoustic energy. To date, several therapeutic substances, such as chemotherapeutics, antibodies, plasmids and viral vectors, have successfully been delivered to the CNS by FUS-induced BBB opening in animal models, including non-human primates. Translation to a clinical application is pending.

Introduction

The blood-brain barrier (BBB) is a highly specialised system separating the vasculature from the intracerebral parenchymal compartment. By preventing the unrestricted entrance of most molecular substances, the BBB protects the brain from potentially harmful substances in the bloodstream. This function is mediated by a complex interplay of specialised endothelial cells, the basal lamina supporting the abluminal surface of the endothelium and astrocytic endfeet attached to the basal lamina. The microvasculature of the central nervous system (CNS) can be distinguished from peripheral tissue endothelial cells by unique characteristics: adjacent endothelial cells are coupled by a continuous network of tight junctions with high electrical resistance, thus 'sealing' the paracellular pathway [1]. Furthermore, CNS endothelial cells lack fenestrations and have very few pinocytotic vesicles, indicating a restricted transcellular passage. Instead, these cells are rich in mitochondria, which are required for active transport of nutrients to the brain from the blood.

Whether a particular substance is capable of crossing the intact BBB depends on several factors, including the molecular weight and size, conformation, amino acid composition and lipophilicity of the molecule, amongst others. Small lipid-soluble molecules up to a molecular mass of about 400 Da can cross the BBB by lipid-mediated free diffusion. Small or large water-soluble molecules need catalysed transport systems such as carrier-mediated transport, active efflux transport and receptor-mediated transcytosis [2]. However, neither carrier-mediated transport systems nor active efflux transport systems permit the delivery of large-molecule drugs. Most of the current potential therapeutic substances, such as chemotherapeutic agents, monoclonal antibodies, recombinant proteins, antisense RNA or gene therapeutics, do not cross the intact BBB and are not substrates of the physiologically active transport systems.

Thus, a variety of methods have been explored to overcome the BBB for facilitation of drug delivery to the CNS, but none have achieved clinical applicability.

The first observations that ultrasound (US) can alter the permeability of the BBB date back to the 1950s. Bakay and colleagues found that focused ultrasound (FUS) applied to cat brains could induce microlesions with severe parenchymal damage, but this technique could also induce transient opening of the BBB, with leakage of Trypan blue lasting around 72 hours [3]. In contrast, the application of unfocused US was followed by distinct extravasation of blue dye and signs of haemorrhage but no relevant damage to the CNS parenchyma [4]. After almost half a century without further development of this technique, Hynynen and colleagues renewed interest in this exciting potential with their results on BBB opening using US approximately one decade ago [5]. Since then, extensive efforts have been undertaken to characterise the mechanisms, the potential side effects and safety aspects as well as the potential clinical applications of FUS-induced BBB opening. This article will give an overview of the mechanisms, the potential side effects as well as the diagnostic and therapeutic applications of US-induced BBB opening.

Mechanisms of Ultrasound-Induced Blood-Brain Barrier Opening

To date, the exact mechanism of US-induced BBB disruption is still not fully understood. In the presence of microbubbles, which serve as preformed cavitation nuclei, both stable and inertial cavitation can contribute to BBB opening [6]. In the case of stable cavitation, the US waves cause bubbles to repeatedly expand and contract, resulting in microstreaming and shear stress on the vessel wall. This effect could, in turn, affect the integrity of the tight junctions of the vessel wall. Inertial cavitation is characterised by violent collapse of the bubbles, and the released energy generates localised shock waves and fluid jets. These mechanical effects may induce BBB opening but can also damage the surrounding tissue, especially at high-pressure amplitudes. Whether stable or inertial cavitation occurs depends on both the peak rarefactional pressure and the diameter of the microbubbles. In mice, the threshold of inertial cavitation during BBB opening was found to be a peak-negative pressure of 0.45 MPa [6]. Peak-negative pressures of 0.15 MPa did not result in BBB opening, while phantom and in vivo studies indicated that BBB opening at 0.15–0.30 MPa in the presence of 4–5-μm microbubbles may occur by stable cavitation alone. However, for small-sized microbubbles with a diameter of 1–2 μm, the identified threshold fell between 0.30–0.45 MPa [7].

Avenues of Transcapillary Passage

The cellular mechanisms of BBB opening are being investigated and may involve several routes. Electron microscopy of rabbits subjected to US-induced BBB disruption showed an increased number of vesicles and vacuoles in the sonicated areas, indicating a possible passage via transcytosis. Furthermore, transendothelial openings in the form of fenestrae-like formations and cytoplasmic channels have been demonstrated [8]. The electron microscopic findings of widened interendothelial clefts with missing zonulae occludentes are supported by immunoelectron microscopy: 1 h after US-induced BBB disruption in rats, the immunosignals for the tight junctional proteins Occludin, Claudin-5 and ZO-1 were markedly reduced. Twenty-four hours after sonication, the density and localisation of the immunosignals appeared to be completely restored. These data indicate that a transient disintegration of the tight junctions, enabling paracellular passage of substances, might be the most important route in US-induced BBB opening [9]. An example of successful opening of the BBB in rats is shown in figure 1.

Extent and Duration of Blood-Brain Barrier Opening

While transcytotic passage is size-independent, as the index agents are carried in cellular vesicles, the paracellular pathway is size-selective. To assess the maximum gap between endothelial cells following US-induced BBB opening, the passage of several magnetic resonance (MR) contrast agents with varying hydrodynamic diameters has been investigated in a rat model. In contrast to smaller-sized contrast agents, the penetration of a 65-nm superparamagnetic contrast agent was limited to the focal point of the transducer, indicating a particle size close to the maximum gap [10]. These results are in accordance with drug-delivery studies, showing successful penetration of macromolecules such as Herceptin [11] (148 kDa, 10 nm) or antibodies [12] as a consequence of US-induced BBB disruption.

The duration of an effective passage following US-induced BBB opening depends mainly on the hydrodynamic diameter of the delivered substances [10]. Small-sized particles of about 1 nm have been shown to cross the BBB over several hours, with full restoration of BBB function at about 24 h. Instead, 4-nm particles only penetrated the BBB 2 h post BBB disruption. A recent analysis predicts that BBB closure dynamics is a function of the hydrodynamic diameter [10].

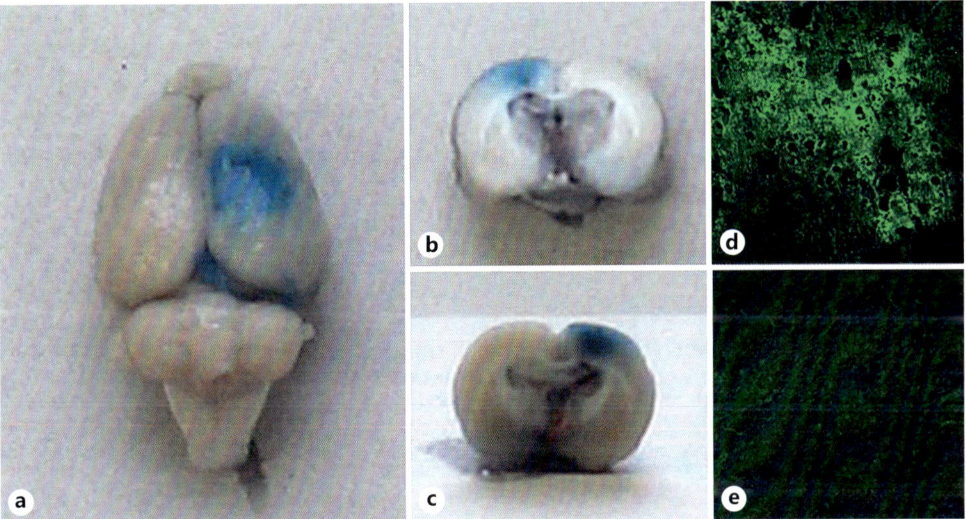

Fig. 1. BBB opening in the rat brain. The right hemisphere was insonicated with focused ultrasound for BBB opening (intracranial pressure amplitude, 1.25 MPa; Optison, 0.1 ml/kg). Macroscopic inspection showed a localised extravasation of Evan's Blue dye on the brain surface (**a**) that penetrated into the underlying cortex (**b**, front side; **c**, reverse side). Immunofluorescence microscopy using antibodies against albumin documented confluent and widespread albumin-positive reaction products in the brain parenchyma of insonicated hemispheres (**d**), while no albumin extravasation was observed in the non-treated left hemisphere (**e**) [30]. Magnification in **d**, **e**: ×200 (taken from Alonso et al. [30]).

Safety Aspects and Side Effects

The first observations of US-induced BBB opening included the detection of microlesions with severe parenchymal damage [3]. Since then, multiple efforts have been undertaken to optimise the US parameters in order to increase the safety of this method. The risk of tissue damage depends on several factors, most importantly the presence of microbubbles and the acoustic energy.

Microbubbles
The introduction of microbubbles, which serve as cavitation nuclei, into the blood stream reduces the US intensity that is needed to produce BBB opening. Thus, the US effects can be confined to the vasculature, diminishing the risk of irreversible neuronal damage.

In the presence of intravenously administered Optison, albumin-coated, octafluoropropan-filled microbubbles with a diameter of about 3–4.5 μm, a focal opening of the BBB could be achieved with negligible damage to the vasculature and surrounding tissue [5].

However, the risk of tissue damage has been shown to increase with increasing microbubble concentration. In a recent study using SonoVue, phospholipid-coated microbubbles with a mean diameter of 2.5 µm, insonation of the rat brain at pressure amplitudes of 1.2 MPa in combination with microbubbles at a low dose (30 µl/kg) did not result in neuronal damage. However, increasing the microbubble dose to 60 µl/kg led to the appearance of apoptotic cells together with augmented extravasation of erythrocytes [13]. To date, there have been no comparisons of the effect of different microbubble formulations on neuronal tissue damage. In a rat model of myocardial contrast echocardiography, the impact of three different contrast agents on vascular permeability has been evaluated, but no significant differences between the microbubbles' microvascular damage potentials were found. These data suggest that shell type and encapsulated gas may have little influence on the bioeffects of microbubbles [14].

Acoustic Energy

Much evidence substantiates the fact that increasing pressure amplitudes are associated with an increased risk of brain tissue damage, with an overlap between feasibility parameters enabling BBB opening and safety parameters ensuring the absence of cell or tissue damage. In mice submitted to sonication at a frequency of 1.525 MHz, the pressure threshold for damage, as detected microscopically in haematoxylin and eosin-stained brain slices, is about 0.6 MPa, while pressure amplitudes of 0.8 MPa led to large-scale haemorrhage [15]. In contrast, pulsed US exposures using a frequency of 1.63 MHz and pressure amplitudes ranging from 0.7 to 1.0 MPa in the brains of rabbits resulted in minor effects on the vasculature but only limited signs of neuronal apoptosis or ischaemia in the sonicated areas [16]. A recent study aiming to identify a safety profile for US-induced BBB opening in the presence of Definity microbubbles in rhesus macaques showed a 50% risk of tissue damage at a frequency of 220 kHz and pressure amplitude of 0.3 MPa.

The different pressure threshold values reported in these and further studies are most likely attributable to several factors. First, anatomical differences between small animals and primates may determine a species-specific damage threshold. Second, acoustic parameters other than the pressure, such as pulse length or frequency, may contribute to the transmitted acoustic energy and thus to possible US-induced tissue damage. Third, there is no consensus as to how 'tissue damage' should be defined and assessed. MR imaging is commonly used to detect haemorrhage but has a rather low sensitivity compared to microscopic evaluation of histological slices. In addition, the time point of evaluation plays an important role, as extravasation of erythrocytes is an early sign of damage, while apoptosis may occur in a delayed fashion.

Accidental Blood-Brain Barrier Opening with Diagnostic Ultrasound?

To investigate the effect of diagnostic transcranial, color-coded sonography on the integrity of the BBB in humans, contrast-enhanced MRI with gadolinium (Gd) was performed in healthy male volunteers following ultrasonic contrast agent destruction of two US contrast agents (Levovist and Optison) [17]. The US parameters were kept within diagnostic limits, with acoustic pressure amplitudes of less than 2.69 MPa, and were attenuated by the temporal bone. Contrast-enhanced MRI with Gd did not show any detectable differences in T1 signal intensities before, immediately after or 2 h after insonation in two defined brain regions, suggesting that the exposure levels of the current ultrasonic equipment do not cause accidental BBB opening. However, more subtle changes to the integrity of the BBB might have been missed due to the relatively large molecular weight of the Gd tracer.

Magnetic Resonance-Guided Focused Ultrasound for Blood Brain Barrier Opening: Advanced Neuroimaging

Since the first systematic studies on US-induced BBB opening by Hynynen and colleagues in 2001 [5], MRI has been widely used to monitor this procedure. MR guidance using contrast-enhanced high-resolution MRI at 9.4 T allowed specific targeting of small anatomical regions, such as the murine hippocampus, as well as a temporal analysis of BBB opening kinetics through repeated Gd-enhanced imaging [18]. Recent work has focused on the potential of non-invasive BBB opening to facilitate MR molecular neuroimaging. In a transgenic mouse model of Alzheimer's disease, US-induced BBB disruption was used to enable molecular imaging of amyloid plaques [12]. The distribution of rabbit anti-Aβ-antibodies given intravenously immediately before FUS was examined immunohistochemically in serial brain sections. Within the transducer focus, enhanced staining was predominantly found around large blood vessels, possibly indicating a limited diffusion of antibodies into the brain parenchyma. Liao and colleagues designed albumin-shelled gadolinium-diethylene triamine pentaacetic acid (albumin-(Gd-DTPA)) microbubbles as a dual modality contrast agent for US and MR imaging [19]. In vitro, the application of albumin-(Gd-DTPA) microbubbles resulted in a significant enhancement of the US contrast in $T(1)$-, $T(2)$- and $T(2)^*$-weighted MR images. In vivo, albumin-(Gd-DTPA) microbubbles did not leak into the brain parenchyma of rats during US-induced BBB opening due to their relatively large size. In contrast, BBB opening accompanying intracranial haemorrhage was characterised by significant leakage of albumin-(Gd-DTPA) microbubbles, making them a useful tool for differentiating focused-US-induced BBB opening from intracranial haemorrhage.

Improved penetration of MR contrast agents for advanced neuroimaging was also achieved with unfocused US, promoting a global, transient disruption of the BBB. In a transgenic mouse model of amyloidosis, the MR contrast agent Gd was injected intravenously after transient opening of the BBB with 1 MHz unfocused US, allowing the high-resolution detection of amyloid plaques with a short imaging time [20]. Unfocused US-induced BBB opening has also been investigated to perform activation-induced, manganese-enhanced MRI in mice [21]. Accumulation of manganese in depolarised neurons in response to mechanical stimulation of the vibrissae was used to generate a functional map of the barrel field cortex.

Delivery of Therapeutic Substances

The intact BBB prevents the entry of most therapeutic substances into the brain. In concrete terms, almost 100% of large-molecule drugs and up to 95% of small-molecule drugs do not cross the BBB [22]. Consequently, US-induced BBB opening offers new perspectives for a broad range of neurotherapeutics. The first investigations on enhanced drug delivery following US-induced BBB opening trace back to Treat and colleagues, who analysed the targeted delivery of the chemotherapeutic drug doxorubicin (DOX) to the rat brain [23]. Using FUS in combination with Optison, local tissue concentrations of DOX exceeding the clinical benchmarks described in previous studies could be achieved with minimal tissue effects. In contrast, the DOX concentration in non-sonicated tissue remained low, thus minimising the risk of neurotoxic effects by DOX. In line with these results, the chemotherapeutic agent cytarabine has successfully been delivered to the rat brain after systemic administration via US-induced BBB opening [24]. The delivery of chemotherapeutics has also been analysed in rodent disease models. Fisher rats implanted with 9L glioma cells were treated with oral temozolomide (TMZ) alone at different doses or in combination with MRI-monitored FUS with microbubbles (TMZ/FUS) [25]. Quantification of TMZ revealed an increased CSF/plasma ratio of TMZ in the TMZ/FUS group. Furthermore, US-enhanced delivery of TMZ significantly suppressed tumour growth, with a reduced 7-day tumour progression ratio, resulting in a prolonged median survival time. In the context of oncological therapy, Kinoshita and colleagues investigated the delivery of antibody-based anticancer agents [11]. The humanised anti-human epidermal growth factor receptor 2 monoclonal antibody trastuzumab, which has been effective in local and distal tumour control in patients with breast cancer, was injected, either alone or in combination with FUS/microbubbles, into the tail vein of mice. As trastuzumab cannot penetrate the intact BBB, the amount of trastuzumab in the non-sonicated tissues was below the detection threshold. In contrast, FUS-induced BBB led to a significant increase of trastuzumab in the target region, with a positive correlation between trastuzumab concentration and the applied acoustic pressure.

To achieve a more sustained therapeutic effect, delivery of genes into the brain, which results in stable expression of the target agent, is appealing. For this purpose, plasmid DNA has been conjugated to the surface of lipid-shelled microbubbles. In mice, intravenous injection of pBDNF-EGFP-loaded microbubbles together with MRI-guided FUS (1.1-MHz transducer; acoustic power, 2.2 W) was followed by internalisation of plasmid DNA into the cytoplasm of neurons in the target region after 1 h. The presence of numerous transparent vesicles in the cytoplasm of these cells suggested a predominantly transcellular passage. Forty-eight hours after transfection, the expression of BDNF was markedly enhanced compared to a control group [26]. A main limitation of gene transfer with plasmid vectors is a rather low level of transfection and subsequent gene expression. In contrast, gene transfer using recombinant adeno-associated virus vectors facilitates stable, long-term, enhanced gene expression. As most viral vectors cannot cross the intact BBB, a combination strategy with US-induced BBB opening has been recently investigated. Chimeric adeno-associated virus 2/1 particles containing the coding region for the LacZ gene were administered intravenously to rats. Upon FUS-induced BBB using a 500-kHz transducer at an effective pressure amplitude of 1 MPa in the presence of microbubbles, the transgene was correctly and efficiently expressed predominantly in neurons within the target region [27].

Recent work suggests that even very large particles, such as stem cells with a mean diameter of 10 μm, may be delivered to the brain via FUS-induced BBB opening. GFP-transfected embryonic cortical neuronal progenitor cells, together with extravasated red blood cells, were found in the sonicated hemisphere of rats 24 h after US treatment [28]. However, further work is needed to exclude long-term damage from this method.

Ultrasound-Induced Blood-Brain Barrier Opening in Primates

When transferring the results from US-induced BBB opening from rodent models to primates, several issues have to be considered. First, attenuation of the US energy through the human skull has to be regarded. Second, internal reflections of the US waves and generation of standing waves, especially at low frequencies, may lead to intracranial haemorrhage. Third, side effects beyond histologically detectable damage and rough neurological deficits cannot be sufficiently deduced from small animal models. In particular, behavioural and cognitive alterations following (repeated) sonications need careful observation in larger animal models before clinical translation.

A recent study by McDannold and colleagues [29] investigated the safety and efficacy of MR-guided, US-induced BBB opening in rhesus macaques using the ExAblate 4000 low-frequency TcMRgFUS System that has been designed for human use. Sonications at a frequency of 220 kHz were performed at a range of pressure amplitudes in 4 rhesus macaques, resulting in a probability of 50% for BBB opening at 149 kPa, and a 50% probability for tissue damage was estimated at 300 kPa. Functional testing in 3 other macaques following repeated sonications of the lateral geniculate nucleus and the visual cortex did not reveal any deficits. Although these results may suggest a relatively 'safe window' given the correct sonication parameters, the authors also found substantial variations of BBB disruption from location-to-location, possibly as a consequence of skull irregularities or different anatomical susceptibility to US-induced BBB opening.

Conclusions

FUS-induced BBB opening is a promising new strategy for overcoming the BBB for treatment of various CNS diseases, including neurodegenerative and genetic disorders, brain tumours and cerebrovascular diseases. In several animal models, including non-human primates, the feasibility of this method has unequivocally been proven. Critical evaluation of the side effects, especially the long-term effects, and possible neuropsychological alterations is indispensable when proceeding towards clinical application in humans.

References

1 Luissint AC, Artus C, Glacial F, et al: Tight junctions at the blood brain barrier: physiological architecture and disease-associated dysregulation. Fluids Barriers CNS 2012;9:23.

2 Pardridge WM: Drug and gene targeting to the brain with molecular Trojan horses. Nat Rev Drug Discov 2002;1:131–139.

3 Bakay L, Ballantine HT Jr, Hueter TF, et al: Ultrasonically produced changes in the blood-brain barrier. Arch NeurPsych 1956;76:457–467.

4 Ballantine HT Jr, Bell E, Manlapaz J: Progress and problems in the neurological applications of focused ultrasound. J Neurosurg 1960;17:858–876.

5 Hynynen K, McDannold N, Vykhodtseva N, et al: Noninvasive MR imaging-guided focal opening of the blood-brain barrier in rabbits. Radiology 2001; 220:640–646.

6 Tung YS, Vlachos F, Choi JJ, et al: In vivo transcranial cavitation threshold detection during ultrasound-induced blood-brain barrier opening in mice. Phys Med Biol 2010;55:6141–6155.

7 Choi JJ, Feshitan JA, Baseri B, et al: Microbubble-size dependence of focused ultrasound-induced blood-brain barrier opening in mice in vivo. IEEE Trans Biomed Eng 2010;57:145–154.

8 Sheikov N, McDannold N, Vykhodtseva N, et al: Cellular mechanisms of the blood-brain barrier opening induced by ultrasound in presence of microbubbles. Ultrasound Med Biol 2004;30:979–989.

9 Sheikov N, McDannold N, Sharma S, et al: Effect of focused ultrasound applied with an ultrasound contrast agent on the tight junctional integrity of the brain microvascular endothelium. Ultrasound Med Biol 2008;34:1093–1104.

10 Marty B, Larrat B, Van Landeghem M, et al: Dynamic study of blood-brain barrier closure after its disruption using ultrasound: a quantitative analysis. J Cereb Blood Flow Metab 2012;32:1948–1958.

11 Kinoshita M, McDannold N, Jolesz FA, et al: Noninvasive localized delivery of Herceptin to the mouse brain by MRI-guided focused ultrasound-induced blood-brain barrier disruption. Proc Natl Acad Sci U S A 2006;103:11719–11723.

12 Raymond SB, Treat LH, Dewey JD, et al: Ultrasound enhanced delivery of molecular imaging and therapeutic agents in Alzheimer's disease mouse models. PLoS One 2008;3:e2175.

13 Yang FY, Fu WM, Yang RS, et al: Quantitative evaluation of focused ultrasound with a contrast agent on blood-brain barrier disruption. Ultrasound Med Biol 2007;33:1421–1427.

14 Li P, Armstrong WF, Miller DL: Impact of myocardial contrast echocardiography on vascular permeability: comparison of three different contrast agents. Ultrasound Med Biol 2004;30:83–91.

15 Baseri B, Choi JJ, Tung YS, et al: Multi-modality safety assessment of blood-brain barrier opening using focused ultrasound and definity microbubbles: a short-term study. Ultrasound Med Biol 2010;36: 1445–1459.

16 McDannold N, Vykhodtseva N, Raymond S, et al: MRI-guided targeted blood-brain barrier disruption with focused ultrasound: histological findings in rabbits. Ultrasound Med Biol 2005;31:1527–1537.

17 Schlachetzki F, Hölscher T, Koch HJ, et al: Observation on the integrity of the blood-brain barrier after microbubble destruction by diagnostic transcranial color-coded sonography. J Ultrasound Med 2002;21: 419–429.

18 Choi JJ, Pernot M, Brown TR, et al: Spatio-temporal analysis of molecular delivery through the blood-brain barrier using focused ultrasound. Phys Med Biol 2007;52:5509–5530.

19 Liao AH, Liu HL, Su CH, et al: Paramagnetic perfluorocarbon-filled albumin-(Gd-DTPA) microbubbles for the induction of focused-ultrasound-induced blood-brain barrier opening and concurrent MR and ultrasound imaging. Phys Med Biol 2012;57:2787–2802.

20 Santin MD, Debeir T, Bridal SL, et al: Fast in vivo imaging of amyloid plaques using μ-MRI Gd-staining combined with ultrasound-induced blood-brain barrier opening. Neuroimage 2013;79:288–294.

21 Howles GP, Qi Y, Johnson GA: Ultrasonic disruption of the blood-brain barrier enables in vivo functional mapping of the mouse barrel field cortex with manganese-enhanced MRI. Neuroimage 2010;50:1464–1471.

22 Pardridge WM: The blood-brain barrier: bottleneck in brain drug development. NeuroRx 2005;2:3–14.

23 Treat LH, McDannold N, Vykhodtseva N, et al: Targeted delivery of doxorubicin to the rat brain at therapeutic levels using MRI-guided focused ultrasound. Int J Cancer 2007;121:901–907.

24 Zeng HQ, Lü L, Wang F, et al: Focused ultrasound-induced blood-brain barrier disruption enhances the delivery of cytarabine to the rat brain. J Chemother 2012;24:358–363.

25 Wei KC, Chu PC, Wang HY, et al: Focused ultrasound-induced blood-brain barrier opening to enhance temozolomide delivery for glioblastoma treatment: a preclinical study. PLoS One 2013;8:e58995.

26. Huang Q, Deng J, Wang F, et al: Targeted gene delivery to the mouse brain by MRI-guided focused ultrasound-induced blood-brain barrier disruption. Exp Neurol 2012;233:350–356.

27 Alonso A, Reinz E, Leuchs B, et al: Focal delivery of AAV2/1-transgenes into the rat brain by localized ultrasound-induced BBB opening. Mol Ther Nucleic Acids 2013;2:e73.

28 Burgess A, Ayala-Grosso CA, Ganguly M, et al: Targeted delivery of neural stem cells to the brain using MRI-guided focused ultrasound to disrupt the blood-brain barrier. PLoS One 2011;6:e27877.

29 McDannold N, Arvanitis CD, Vykhodtseva N, et al: Temporary disruption of the blood-brain barrier by use of ultrasound and microbubbles: safety and efficacy evaluation in rhesus macaques. Cancer Res 2012;72:3652–3663.

30 Alonso A, Reinz E, Jenne JW, Fatar M, Schmidt-Glenewinkel H, Hennerici MG, Meairs S: Reorganization of gap junctions after focused ultrasound blood-brain barrier opening in the rat brain. J Cereb Blood Flow Metab 2010;30:1394–1402.

PD Dr. Angelika Alonso
Department of Neurology
Universitätsmedizin Mannheim, University of Heidelberg
Theodor-Kutzer-Ufer 1–3, DE–68167 Mannheim (Germany)
E-Mail alonso@neuro.ma.uni-heidelberg.de

Author Index

Subject Index